HOW THE WORLD WORKS
MEDICINE

D1020989

HOW THE WORLD WORKS
MEDICINE

From early healing to the miracles of modern medicine

Anne Rooney

ARCTURUS

With thanks to Bill Thompson, for patience, support and coffee.

PICTURE CREDITS – Andrew Weston: 186. **Bridgeman Art Library:** 28, 42, 51, 100, 116 (top), 132, 134, 148 (left), 150, 152 (top), 164, 183. **clipart.com:** 48, 49 (top), 54 (left), 60, 66 (bottom), 69, 75 (top), 78, 81, 91 (bottom), 99 (bottom), 102 (top), 115, 120, 131 (bottom), 145 (bottom), 152 (bottom), 160 (bottom right), 167, 200. **Corbis:** 9, 25, 38, 40 (top), 44, 50, 62 (bottom), 63, 93 (bottom), 128, 165. **John Campana:** 166. **Library of Congress:** 149 (top). **Mary Evans:** 31, 49 (bottom), 57, 64 (left), 73 (top), 77 (bottom), 84, 105, 122 (bottom), 125, 130, 139 (top), 140, 156 (bottom), 158, 185, 190, 197 (bottom), 198. **Photos.com:** 8, 16, 19 (top), 27, 30, 34, 39 (bottom), 72, 112, 119, 143 (bottom), 154, 157 (bottom), 193 (top). **Picture Desk: Kobal Collection:** 199. **Rebecca Glover:** 19 (bottom), 22 (left), 62 (top). **Science Photo Library:** 13, 18 (bottom), 33 (top), 36, 46, 61 (left), 64 (right), 68, 70 (right), 73 (bottom), 80 (right), 90, 95 (bottom), 122 (top), 123, 138 (top), 141, 142 (top), 146 (top), 151 (bottom), 160 (bottom left), 170, 172 (bottom), 178, 184, 187, 188, 196 (all), 202 (bottom). **Shutterstock:** 6, 7, 12, 14 (bottom), 21 (top), 45 (top), 64 (bottom), 71 (right), 74 (left), 76, 78 (bottom), 83, 88 (top), 95 (top), 97 (all), 98 (bottom), 99 (top left),102 (bottom), 110, 113 (bottom), 114 (bottom), 118 (top), 133 (top), 138 (bottom), 197 (left), 204. **Topfoto:** 14 (top), 37 (bottom), 41, 52 (bottom), 96 (top), 108, 131 (top), 137, 146 (bottom), 153, 155, 162, 179. **Wellcome Library:** 135.

ARCTURUS

This edition published in 2017 by Arcturus Publishing Limited
26/27 Bickels Yard, 151–153 Bermondsey Street,
London SE1 3HA

Copyright © Arcturus Holdings Limited

All rights reserved. No part of this publication may be reproduced, stored in a retrieval system, or transmitted, in any form or by any means, electronic, mechanical, photocopying, recording or otherwise, without prior written permission in accordance with the provisions of the Copyright Act 1956 (as amended). Any person or persons who do any unauthorised act in relation to this publication may be liable to criminal prosecution and civil claims for damages.

ISBN: 978-1-78428-662-0
AD001081UK

Printed in Malaysia

Contents

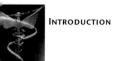

SHORT LIVES AND THE LONG ART

IN SICKNESS AND IN HEALTH

The story of medicine is also the story of disease. It must give voice not only to the scientists and healers who have studied and combated disease and injury, but to the sufferers who have endured illness – and the proddings, pokings and experimentations of medical science.

It is tempting to think that the diseases and accidents that trouble humankind have

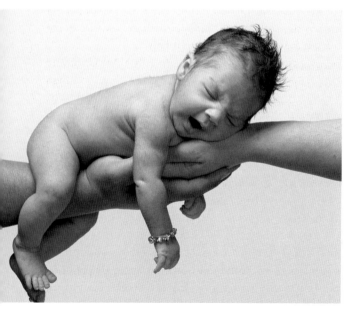

Vital spark: when does life begin? And what creates human consciousness?

always been there, always the same, and only our abilities to deal with them have changed. But it is not so.

Epidemic diseases did not affect our distant forebears. An epidemic needs a reservoir – a population who will harbour the bacterium or virus and allow it to break out periodically in a flurry of new infections. When our ancestors roamed the plains and mountains and the land was sparsely populated, people were too spread out to provide such a reservoir. Contagious and epidemic disease is largely a product of urbanization, when people live in sufficient numbers and sufficiently close proximity to make person-to-person transmission an effective way for a disease to spread.

Nor are human diseases uniquely ours. We share more than sixty disease-inducing micro-organisms with dogs, fifty with cattle, and many with sheep, pigs and poultry.

When hunter-gatherers settled to farming around 12,000 years ago, close contact with animals increased our exposure to the bacteria, viruses and even parasites that preyed on them. Many diseases jumped the species barrier.

We have caught flu from pigs and fowl, colds from horses and measles from dogs or cows. It is not a one-way trade; research in 2008 suggests that tuberculosis in cattle originated in humans, not the other way round (as had been thought for years). It is not even a process that is finished. The emergence in the 1990s of variant Creutzfeld-Jacob disease in people who had eaten beef infected with BSE showed we are not yet off the hook, and the flu virus continues to cross the species barrier. The H1N1 variant which emerged in Mexico in 2009 originated in pigs.

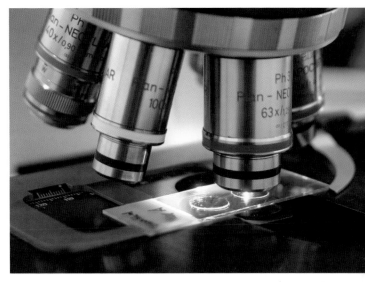

What goes on in the world that is invisible to the naked eye is often crucial to our health – microscopes are a key medical tool

The development of urban societies offered other opportunities for disease. War and trade carried disease to new places. The Romans probably brought bubonic plague to Europe from the east; Spanish conquistadors caught syphilis in their rape of pre-Columbian America, but exchanged it for smallpox, measles and flu which devastated local populations even more quickly than European swords and guns.

While a population that is accustomed to an illness becomes resistant to a degree, a new disease easily wreaks havoc. Eventually, as a society becomes habituated to it, a disease recedes in the general population and restricted to childhood, afflicting those who have not been exposed to it before.

Cities are innately unhealthy. Until very recently, urban death rates were so high that cities could only be sustained by the constant influx of a new population from the countryside.

As well as a population reservoir that can harbour disease, cities have brought new illnesses of their own, arising from urban conditions such as polluted water supplies and overcrowding (cholera and typhoid), poor diet (scurvy), occupation-related disorders and diseases (emphysemia) and conditions brought about by pollution (bronchitis). Most recently, diseases of affluence have clustered in cities – the effects of substance abuse, over-eating and lack of exercise, for example.

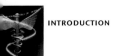

THE FIRST DOCTORS

For as long as there have been sick or injured people, there must have been others trying to help them. For our most distant ancestors, systemic disease was a mystery, often approached with the aid of magic, superstition and religion. Injuries are less mysterious and more easily visible, and also more amenable to simple treatment. Splints and bandages were no doubt used for many thousands of years before we have any record of them. At some point, more than 5,000 years ago in some societies, a form of the medical profession emerged, with particular individuals who specialized in dealing with health problems. In some cases they may have used magical means; in others they used practical methods that were more or less efficacious.

The training of medics began at least 2,500 years ago in Europe, probably longer ago in the Far East. Since that time, we have come to understand much of how the human body works and how it goes wrong; what causes infections and what may cure them; the chemistry that governs life and can cause death. The history of medicine, medics and disease shows humankind coming to understand the bodies we inhabit, developing models for how we work and how diseases affect us. It encompasses the development of medicines, surgery and other interventions, and our attempts to control the innermost workings of the mind and of genetics. And, of course, it includes the histories of the people who have cared for the sick and struggled to extend the boundaries of knowledge.

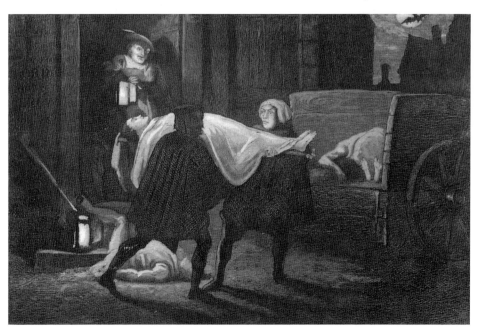

Bring out your dead: a body is taken away for disposal during the Plague of London, 1665. Cities used to be so unhealthy that populations could only be sustained by a constant influx of new blood from the country

To and Fro

The story we will trace here begins in the ancient world. In China, India, Mesopotamia and Egypt, men (for it was mostly men) began to specialize in treating their sick colleagues. They tried to understand how bodies work and how they go wrong, and came up with different models and explanations.

The narratives of Chinese and Indian medicine pursued their own paths, and have diverted little in the last 2,000 years from their original directions. Western medicine has taken a circuitous route from its origins in Mesopotamia and Egypt. The story will take us from Egypt to Ancient Greece, where Hippocrates laid the foundations of modern medicine. From there we follow Hellenic doctors back to Egypt as they filled the hospital of Alexandria, and on to Rome where we meet Galen and Celsus. The rise of Arab culture picked up the legacy of the Greek and Hellenic doctors and fused it with what they learned from Indian, Egyptian and Byzantine medicine to make huge advances of their own. The wisdom of the Arab medics passed back to Europe through Spain and Italy, bringing too the works of the Greeks, lost to Europe for more than a thousand years.

From the Renaissance onwards, western Europe became the focus of advances in medicine. First Italy and then Germany, France and Britain produced medical schools and began a systematic scientific exploration of the human body and its ills. With the Enlightenment, the flourishing of science of all types contributed to medical advances. The new confidence in applying reason, challenging age-old authorities and breaking with traditional taboos and religious prohibitions led to rapid progress. Microscopes, chemistry, electricity, anaesthetics, antisepsis… developments came thick and fast that enabled medicine to advance by leaps and bounds. In just over a hundred years, from 1898 to the present, we have seen the advent of X-rays, microsurgery, transplants, IVF, lasers, robotic telesurgery, genetic engineering and the mapping of the human genome. We can work the magic our ancestors dreamed of, and explain exactly how it functions.

Not Over Yet

Much has been achieved, but the story of medicine is far from finished. We are no closer than the Ancient Greeks to knowing at which point after conception life begins, or understanding what that magic spark is that animates flesh and blood and creates consciousness. We may be able to identify the cause of inherited deformity and disease, but we cannot yet fix genes to prevent its expression. There are diseases we cannot cure and injuries we do not know how to heal. We may wipe out one disease – smallpox – but a host of new ones appears, all just as deadly and incurable: AIDS, Ebola fever, SARS. There is much cause to celebrate the triumphs achieved by the men and women who have battled bravely, tirelessly – and sometimes foolishly – to conquer the ills that flesh is heir to. But there is no room for complacency: when the US Surgeon General said in 1969 that the book of infectious diseases was closed, he was speaking far too soon.

Anne Rooney

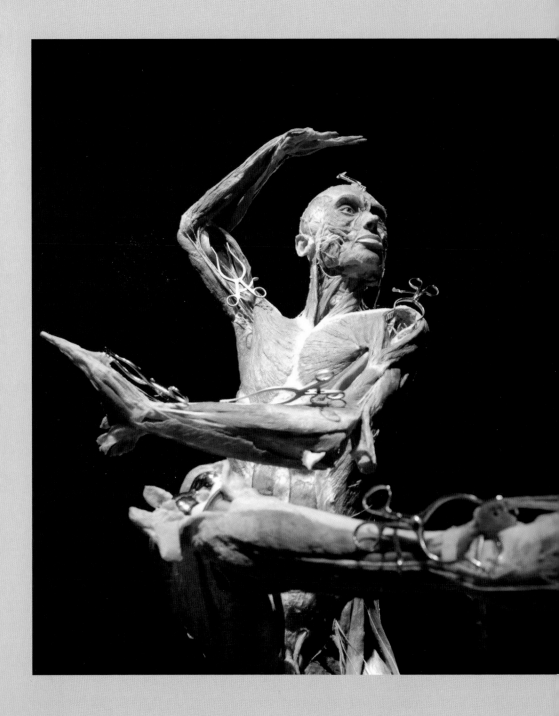

CHAPTER 1

'WHAT A PIECE OF WORK IS A MAN'

The raw material of medicine is the human body and the work of medicine is to maintain the body in perfect condition – or restore it if it goes wrong. This entails knowing how the body should work when it is well. But humankind's concept of the body and how it works has changed radically over time.

The current predominant western view is that the body is an incredibly complex set of finely tuned biochemical systems. But this way of thinking would be completely alien to an ancient Greek proponent of humoral theory. Even modern eastern practitioners are accustomed to thinking in terms of a body that channels energy, and would not recognize the western scientific model. Our present knowledge of the physical and chemical workings of the body has come about through a process of observation, experimentation and examination that has been particularly intense over the last 500 years. It is by no means complete. The path has been tortuous – not least for patients – but the journey of discovery has been a fascinating one.

The workings of the body laid bare in one of Gunther von Hagen's plastinated corpses

On balance

It may seem obvious that it is not possible to gain much knowledge about the human body by looking just at the outside. Yet many societies around the world and throughout history have forbidden making any form of incision in a dead body.

Models of the body have been constructed from what could be observed and deduced from the exterior, from examining injuries and from intellectual models of the world in general. The earliest models of the body focused on balance – whether of energies, elements or 'humours'. Strangely enough, our latest models of the healthy body also feature balance, though of a different type.

There are two broadly different ways of looking at the body and its state of health or illness. One is the holistic and often spiritually-oriented model that is characteristic of eastern philosophies; the other is the atomistic, physically-grounded model that underlies western medicine. This second model only developed once medical scientists were able to take the human body apart and examine its workings, as though they were dismantling an infinitely complex machine. It is a project that is still in progress.

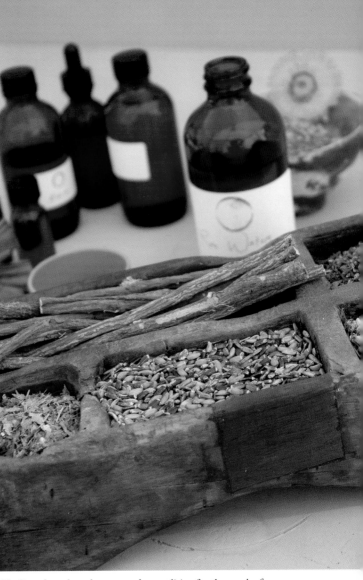

Healing plants have been central to medicine for thousands of years

ENERGY IN THE BALANCE

Eastern medical systems are holistic. That is, they see the body and the spirit as one, governed by flowing and balanced energies. Therapies based around them have developed, evolved and receded, but the central premise that illness is caused by blockages in energy paths or the sluggish flow of energy has remained intact amongst proponents until modern times. This model of illness is very closely related to the spiritual status of the patient, because spiritual and mystical matters affect or dictate the flow of energy. The oldest surviving and continuing medical system is Ayurveda (the Sanskrit word for 'science of life'), which dates from the Vedic age in India – around 3,500 years ago. In China, the oldest and greatest medical text, the *Nei Ching (Canon of Internal Medicine)*, is still studied. It dates perhaps from the 3rd millennium BC, during the reign of Emperor Hwang Ti – and was possibly even written by him. Both Ayurveda and traditional Chinese medicine are still used

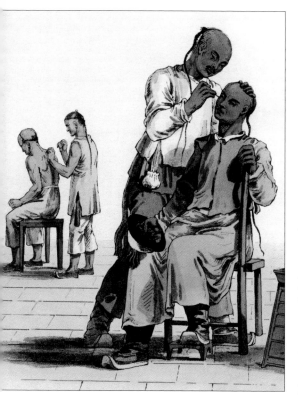

Chinese acupuncture aims to restore the flow of qi *in the patient's body*

by billions of people and the models of the body on which they depend are central to Buddhist and Hindu beliefs.

The medical knowledge at the heart of Ayurveda is said to have been revealed by divine beings. It is preserved in hymn-like verses and its supposedly divine source allows no space for improvement by medical science. Ayurveda teaches that a person should live for around one hundred years, in a state of physical, spiritual and mental wellbeing. This can be achieved by following a healthy lifestyle and responding quickly to signs of illness. The Ayurvedic practitioner treats the body, the mind and the spirit together, aiming to balance the three *doshas* – wind/spirit/air, bile and phlegm – in the body. The correct balance of these is fixed at the moment of conception and maintaining the balance, or returning to one's correct personal balance, is the key to health. Ayurveda uses medicines derived from plants to stimulate the body to rebalance itself. It also makes use of yoga, meditation, massage and, when necessary, surgery.

Qi

Traditional Chinese medicine also ties the physical condition of the body to the health of the spirit. The legendary emperor Shen Nung (approximately 2698BC) is credited with inventing medicine, working with the divine inspiration of the god Pan Ku: the creator, in Taoist tradition. Pan Ku is said to have overcome chaos and to have established the polar principles of yin and yang, which are mingled in all things. Yin is associated with cold, wet, shadow and the female aspect; yang is associated with heat,

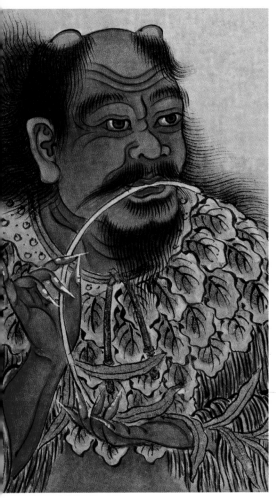

Shen Nung, reputed inventor of medicine in Chinese tradition

the stomach). The organs correspond to 12 main meridian lines. In a healthy body, the yin and the yang organs are in balance, and yin and yang are in balance within individual organs or groups of organs. Any imbalance between the two, whether located in a specific organ or more generally, results in ill health: a 'yang' disease brings about an increase in the body's yang factor and results in a 'hot' disease; a 'yin' disease causes too much yin in the body and a 'cold' disease follows.

The balance and the flow of a special type of energy, called *qi*, is also considered instrumental in determining health or sickness. *Qi* flows easily through the healthy body along meridians, which are not physical conduits but intangible energy pathways. A blockage in the flow of *qi* causes illness; if the flow is seriously impeded, death is inevitable. To restore a healthy flow of *qi* and a balance of yin and

light, dryness and the male aspect. The two necessarily coexist, each defined by its opposite, and are held in balance in a healthy organism or system. In the traditional Chinese model, the body has 12 organs. There are six solid yin organs (such as the heart, the liver and the spleen) and six hollow yang organs (such as the small and large intestine, the bladder and

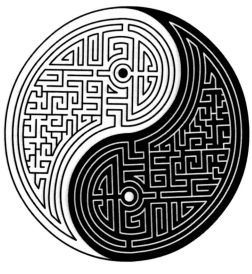

Yin and yang together form a balanced whole

yang, the Chinese doctor uses medicinal plants, massage, special diets, physical exercise regimes or acupuncture.

CHAKRAS

Buddhist and Hindu belief systems formed in India and Tibet teach that the body is governed by many chakras, or energy centres. There are seven major chakras: six are aligned in an ascending column from the base of the spine to the top of the head and one hovers outside the body, between the genitals and the knees. Each chakra is associated with different functions or aspects of consciousness. Chakras are invisible to the human eye, but believers maintain that trained energy workers can perceive them intuitively. They are said to look something like a funnel with petals.

The ideal situation is for the energy that emanates from the chakras low in the body to move upwards. Union with the divine is achieved through the perfect flow of energy from the top of the head. If there is an imbalance or an energy blockage in a chakra then physical or mental illness can result. There are many ways to get recalcitrant chakras back in order, including using special stones and chanting. Yoga, too, is said to open the chakras and encourage the flow of energy, helping to maintain health. In addition, each individual is said to have an aura, something like a border of energy around the body. It is considered important to keep the aura clean, because it can be polluted by foreign and negative energies and vibrations. Methods of cleaning the aura include dusting the space around the body with an owl feather, combing the space with the fingers, standing under a waterfall or – more banally – bathing in Epsom salts.

THE FOUR HUMOURS

From the 5th century BC until the 19th century, the predominant model of the body in Europe and the Middle East was of a vessel composed of four humours that had to be kept in balance if good health was to be maintained. The humours were black bile, yellow bile, blood and phlegm. Too much or too little of any one of these humours would lead to illness, which must be treated by restoring balance. The body was encouraged to produce more of the unbalanced humour, or expel the excess. The origins of humoral theory probably lie in Mesopotamia or Egypt, but the concept was developed in classical Greece. It survived for two millennia, associated largely with the great Greek doctor Hippocrates (see p.18). The humours were related to the four elements – fire, earth, air and water – from which, according to Pythagoras and Empedocles, everything on earth was created. These were combined with the elemental pairs of opposites identified by Alcmaeon: hot and cold, wet and dry, sweet and sour, and so on. Alcmaeon thought that health depended on the balance between these opposites. He used a political metaphor to define health and disease: if the opposing powers are balanced, the body is healthy, but if any one becomes king, disease results. Sources of imbalance included the environment, diet, climate and internal factors. Alcmaeon's model did not require any recourse to the supernatural or the mystical, but suggested that the patient could be healed without

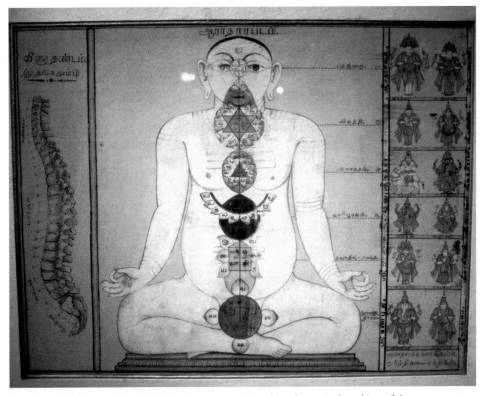

In traditional Indian medicine, six chakras (energy centres) are located at major branchings of the nervous system

the intervention of the divine, simply by restoring the disturbed balance.

Humoral theory was concerned with mental health and temperament as well as with physical wellbeing. This aspect of humorism was first developed by the Graeco-Roman doctor Galen (AD129–c.216), one of the most influential figures in the history of medicine (see p.22), and later by the 11th-century Arab doctor Avicenna. Like Hippocrates, Galen believed that health required a balance of the four humours, but he went further by asserting that there could be an imbalance of humours in an individual organ which could lead to a local disorder. After Hippocrates

and Galen, diseases were categorized and treated according to the particular humoral imbalance that was thought to produce them. Different temperaments and proportions of humours were believed to be natural at different stages of life; old people would incline towards a cold, dry condition, while young people would be hot and moist. This helped to explain why some diseases were common at certain stages of a person's life. An old person might be prone to arthritis, rheumatism and other cold, moist conditions, for instance. The nature and cure of a disease depended on its humoral qualities – so leprosy, a cold disease, must be treated with heat.

ALCMAEON

Alcmaeon, a contemporary of Pythagoras, was associated with the medical school at Croton in the 5th century BC. He was one of the pioneers of Greek rational medicine, which set the foundation for the whole of western medicine. Alcmaeon recognized the brain as the seat of the intellect and the senses and suggested that it was connected to the sensory organs by channels (*poroi*). He discovered the Eustachian tube in the ear, he distinguished arteries from veins, he possibly found the optic nerve and he described a model of vision based on external light, internal fire and liquid in the eyes. His theory that sleep and death result from the partial or complete ebbing of blood from the brain was accepted until the beginning of the 20th century.

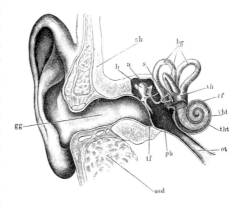

Alcmaeon discovered the Eustachian tube (ot) which links the pharynx to the middle ear

It was thought that minor variations in the ratio of humours accounted for differences of personality and temperament and that this personal balance might also make a person particularly susceptible to certain diseases. According to this model, a person with too much blood would be sanguine (courageous and hopeful) and a person with too much black bile would be melancholic (depressive and irritable). This type of imbalance of the humours, if severe, was often considered to be hereditary and beyond hope of cure.

The humoral model passed from the Greeks to the Romans and later dominated Byzantine medicine. In around 850, the Arab physician Hunayn ibn Ishaq listed 129 works by Galen that had been translated into Arabic or Syriac, revealing the extent to which his influence was already felt. Some

Humour	Element	Nature	Conditions
Black bile	Earth	Cold and dry	Depressive, insomniac, irritable
Blood	Air	Warm and moist	Courageous, hopeful, amorous
Phlegm	Water	Cold and moist	Unemotional, calm, phlegmatic
Yellow bile	Fire	Warm and dry	Bad-tempered, quick to anger

HIPPOCRATES (c.460–c.375BC)

Hippocrates is lauded as the father of modern medicine – the giant on whose shoulders all western physicians have stood. Despite his mythic stature, relatively little is known about his life and works and there is no near-contemporary account of him. He was born on the Greek island of Kos in around 450 or 460BC, where he learned medicine from his father, a physician. After travelling widely around Greece he returned to Kos and taught for many years at the medical school there. He had a deep understanding of and sympathy for the suffering of the sick, and made the care of the patient central to his philosophy.

Hippocrates rejected divine intervention as a source of disease or healing and instead developed diagnostic practices based on observation and reason. Human dissection was prohibited in ancient Greece so he had to base his anatomical knowledge on the dissection of animals and the pathology of sick patients. He was unable to make a study of the healthy body for comparative purposes. Hippocrates' name is attached to a body of around 60 texts, which were gathered together in Alexandria about a hundred years after his death, though he probably wrote few of them. They deal with many aspects of medical theory and practice and all are written in a clear, accessible style. The Hippocratic Oath was, according to tradition, originally an oath taken by Hippocrates' own students under a famous plane tree at the medical school. After Hippocrates' death, it is said that honey from the bees on his grave took on miraculous healing powers.

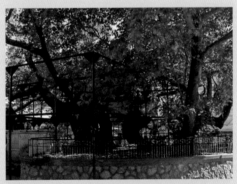

A plane tree on the island of Kos, said to be descended from the one under which Hippocrates taught

Arab doctors began to doubt the validity of the humoral theory. Rhazes (865–925) wrote a text called *Doubts about Galen* in which he declared that taking a hot or cold drink did not automatically alter the temperature of the body. In other words, there was more to it than the simple transfer of heat energy that had been suggested by humoral theory.

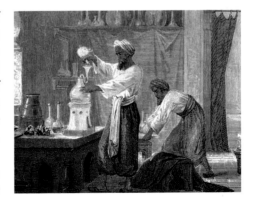

Rhazes busy working on medical concoctions in his laboratory

Avenzoar (1091–1161) discovered that scabies was not caused by humoral imbalance but by a parasite. But nothing was sufficient to discredit Galen completely. Avicenna (c.980–1037) strengthened the stranglehold that humorism held over medicine by refining the relation of the humours to mental and emotional wellbeing in his groundbreaking work on psychology. This aspect of humorism was later explored at length by the English writer Richard Burton in *The Anatomy of Melancholy* (1621), the first comprehensive study of what would now be called clinical depression.

Galen's works entered western Europe in the 11th century in Latin, but they had not been translated directly from the Greek. Instead they were translations of Arab commentaries or Arab versions of Galen's

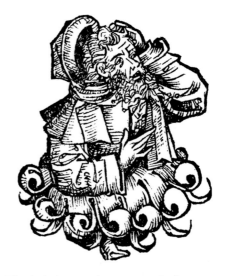

The Arab physician Avenzoar was the first to identify a parasite as the cause of disease

original texts. It was in this second-hand form that Galen's influence was felt in the Middle Ages. From 1490, new translations from Galen's Greek originals appeared and the Greek text itself was published in 1525. A new enthusiasm for Galen's methods, including his practice of undertaking practical investigations, ironically led to his fall from grace as his errors came to light.

Discovering the body's secrets

Little changed in the way that people thought of the human body before the Renaissance.

The balance of humours, or of yin and yang, was considered sufficient explanation of how the body functioned and malfunctioned. All that was to change in the West, but not until people were able for the first time to examine the body in great detail. The Renaissance brought two great developments that would revolutionize our

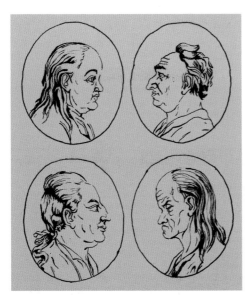

The four humoral temperaments: phlegmatic, choleric, melancholic and sanguine (clockwise from top left)

19

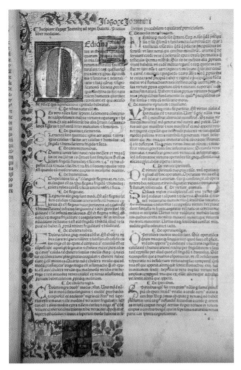

A 13th-century manuscript of the Articella, *documenting a doctor instructing a student*

He advised the researcher to put a dead body into a basket and immerse it in a river for seven days, so that the putrefying flesh would become soft enough to poke away with a stick. The inner organs would then be revealed for inspection. In some cultures, animal dissection supplied anatomical knowledge which was then inappropriately applied to humans. The Egyptian hieroglyph for the womb shows the bipartite uterus of a cow, indicating that doctors had depended on knowledge derived from butchery or ritual sacrifice. The knowledge of human internal organs that embalmers must surely have accrued was apparently not passed to medics. Embalmers were considered unclean and their knowledge was perhaps not thought worthy. Egyptian physicians did, however, take advantage of the opportunities afforded by traumatic injury to take a look inside the body and they recorded their findings. One papyrus describes what a doctor might see inside a crushed skull.

model of the body and change the face of medicine. The first was the beginning of anatomy as a study, based for the first time on the dissection of dead bodies. The second was the invention of the microscope in Holland in the late 16th century.

THE CUTTING EDGE

Many early societies forbade the dissection of human corpses. Neither Indian nor Chinese medicine was based on anatomical knowledge derived from dissection, because it was feared that cutting the body would disadvantage the dead in the afterlife. The Indian surgeon Susruta (6th century BC) managed to bypass the restriction on knives.

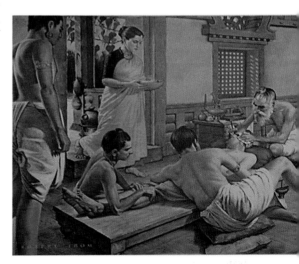

Susruta was a great doctor as well as an anatomist

You find that the smash which is in his skull [is like] the corrugations which appear on [molten] copper in the crucible, and something therein throbs and flutters under your fingers like the weak place in the crown of the head of a child when it has not become whole.

The Greeks, too, shrank from cutting up dead human bodies. Their ideas of the inner structures of the human body are clearly based on studies of animal bodies.

The first anatomists perhaps appeared in Hellenic Alexandria. Herophilos (c.335–260BC) and Erasistratus (304–250BC) are credited with founding the medical school there and carrying out public dissections. Later commentators report that they also carried out vivisection on slaves and condemned prisoners. There are no contemporary records to confirm whether this is true, but the discoveries credited to them make it plausible. Erasistratus was the first experimental physiologist. He investigated the brain and the nerves and suggested that the nerves were hollow tubes that carried a 'nervous spirit' from the brain around the body.

Herophilos, the father of scientific anatomy, also carried out research on the brain, which he recognized as the command centre of the nervous system. He contradicted Aristotle by claiming that the brain is the seat of intelligence. He was the first to distinguish between sensory and motor nerves, and he made the first clear distinction between arteries and veins. Herophilos was also the first physician to measure the pulse, which he did using a water clock. He discovered and named the

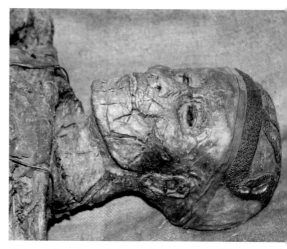

Although Egyptian embalmers removed organs while mummifying bodies, their knowledge was apparently not shared with doctors

duodenum and the prostate, described the function of the nerves and stated that the blood vessels were filled with blood. The latter might seem rather obvious, but earlier doctors believed that the vessels were filled with air. This belief persisted for another 450 years, until Galen demonstrated that it was a fallacy (see p.27).

The Greeks' foray into dissection was short-lived, because the practice was soon banned again. Galen dissected dead animals and experimented on living animals, but he did not extend his experiments and examinations to human subjects. In fact, he made several errors by assuming that human physiology mimicked the animal physiology he had investigated.

Neither the early Christians nor the Muslims allowed the dissection of human corpses. However, the rediscovery of the works of Aristotle in the late 12th century fired a renaissance that embraced the

GALEN (AD129–C.216)

Born in Pergamum, Smyrna (modern Izmir), Galen studied medicine at the greatest medical school of the ancient world, in Alexandria. He worked as chief physician to the gladiators of Pergamum, but then moved to Rome where he served as an army surgeon before attending the emperors Marcus Aurelius, Commodus and Septimius Severus. He advocated dissection and the study of anatomy as the basis of medical knowledge. The dissection of human corpses was forbidden, so his research was confined to work on animals, which distorted his findings and caused him to record a number of errors. Nevertheless, his powers of observation and deduction were considerable. He distinguished between arteries and veins and he worked out the function of several nerves.

Galen was not only a brilliant physician – he was also an accomplished self-publicist and a prolific writer. These skills helped him secure his lasting influence over European and Middle Eastern medicine. His works quickly took over from other texts and dominated Middle Eastern and European medical tradition for centuries.

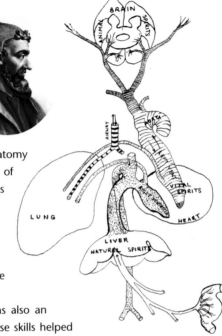

Galen's influential – and enduring – model of the internal workings of the human body

experimental method. Aristotle's work on animals was drawn directly from experiments in vivisection and dissection, which legitimized these practices and paved the way for the reappearance of human dissection. Religion had a role to play here and for once its influence favoured scientific progress. The Fourth Lateran Council of 1215 set out the stance of the Catholic Church on, amongst other things, the nature of resurrection. St Thomas Aquinas (1225–74) explained that on the Day of Judgement the soul and the body would be made whole again – so clearly the body need not be entire for resurrection to take place. Although there is a common belief that the Church prohibited medical dissection or the cutting up of bodies in general, this is not actually the case. During the Crusades, the bodies of several kings and nobles who died far from home were boiled down, or cut up and stored in alcohol, to be transported home for burial – with no fear that this would cost them their chance of

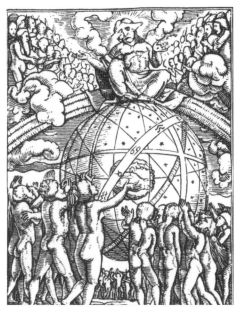

Bodies – even if dissected – will be made whole on Judgement Day according to the medieval church

life in the hereafter. Pope Boniface VIII banned the practice in 1300 because it was disgusting rather than ungodly. There were even cases of the Church directly sanctioning dissection. In the early 13th century, Pope Innocent III ordered a post-mortem examination to discover the cause of a death. And saints were sometimes embalmed, so they had to be cut open.

Dissection was ordered by other authorities, too. In 1302 the first known autopsy was carried out in Bologna, Italy, when a judge ordered the body of a suspected victim of poisoning to be opened. Later on, victims of the Black Death were sometimes dissected.

BODIES PIECEMEAL

Systematic dissection in medical schools began at Salerno in Italy, the first of the European medical schools, in around 1150. At first only pigs were cut up. Dissection soon spread to other Italian schools. In Bologna, Mondino dei' Luzzi (d.1326) became the first doctor to carry out public dissections personally as a teaching aid. He broke with tradition by carrying out the dissection himself, instead of having an assistant do it under his direction. In 1316 he was also the first person to publish a practical manual of anatomy, which was essentially a guide to dissecting a criminal who had been executed by hanging or beheading. He began by making two incisions in the shape of a cross over the abdomen. The dissection examined the contents of three cavities – the abdomen, the thorax and the head. The procedure was little different from modern practice.

Dissections became popular public spectacles in Italy. They were mainly carried out on executed criminals who had lived some distance from the town (30 miles was a common minimum limit). It was often considered the final humiliation and punishment of the criminal, though in 1482 Pope Sixtus IV proclaimed that the dissection of executed criminals must be followed by a proper Christian burial. At the same time, wealthy patients often asked for an autopsy (not a public event) in order to establish the cause of death. There is a record of a family requesting an autopsy in 1502 as a means of establishing the incompetence of the attending physician.

Most dissections were carried out in winter, because the cold weather delayed putrefaction (more a consideration in warm Italy than it would have been in northern Europe). The dissection table was sited in

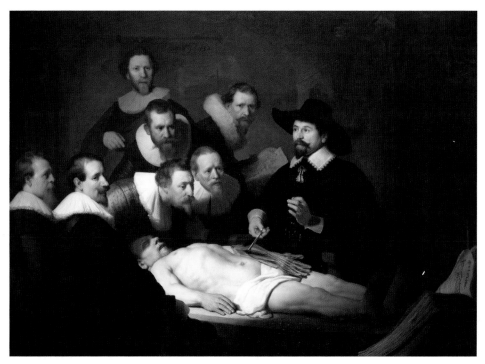

The Anatomy Lesson of Dr Nicolaes Tulp, *Rembrandt, 1632*

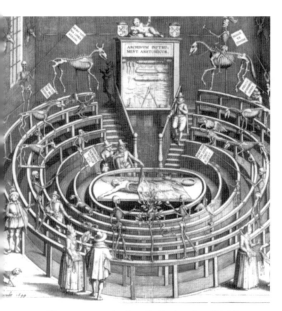

The anatomy school at the University of Leiden

the central well of an amphitheatre. It was surrounded by tiered seating that afforded the audience a good view. Dissections were hardly clinical affairs, as contemporary illustrations reveal.

SUPPLY AND DEMAND

Anatomists needed a constant supply of cadavers to dissect, whether the dissection was intended as a public spectacle or for teaching purposes. The growing demand from medical schools put pressure on the legal supply of bodies. In Great Britain the Murder Act of 1752 allowed the bodies of all executed criminals to be dissected for anatomical research and education. But legal reform during the early decades of the 19th century led to fewer executions, so

THE RESUSCITATION OF ANNE GREEN

Although most people feared that the anatomist's table would become their fate after death, it worked to the benefit of a few. Anne Green was an unfortunate woman who at the age of 22 had given birth prematurely to an illegitimate child which then died.

Whether she had murdered the child or it had died naturally is not clear, but in 1650 she was hanged in Oxford for the baby's murder. Eventually she was cut down and placed in a coffin. She was then passed to three surgeons for dissection. When they opened the coffin, the 'corpse' took a breath. The surgeons made strenuous efforts to revive her and they finally succeeded. She was granted a reprieve by the court, after which she moved to a new life in the countryside, taking her coffin with her.

Edinburgh University, along with items made from his tanned skin. After the murders, British law changed in order to prevent a recurrence. The 1832 Anatomy Act extended the legal supply of corpses so that murder or 'resurrection' should no longer be necessary.

THE GREAT AGE OF THE ANATOMISTS

The anatomists were intent on breaking the human body down into its smallest parts. As a result, the intellectual model of the body began to change. The body was seen to be divided into systems (circulatory, digestive, respiratory and so on), that worked independently as well as together. The first breakthrough came with the work

corpses became scarce. Physicians increasingly turned to body-snatchers (or 'resurrectionists') who stole bodies and then sold them to medical schools.

Between 1827 and 1828 two Irish immigrants, William Burke and William Hare, murdered 17 victims in order to sell their bodies to the University of Edinburgh Medical School. Most of them went to the surgeon Robert Knox. Their first sale was the body of a tenant who had died naturally in Hare's lodging house. They then murdered a sick, elderly tenant by making him drunk and suffocating him. This became their usual *modus operandi* as they lured more people to the boarding house in order to replace their vanishing tenants. Their killing spree continued over a period of 18 months. When they were finally caught, Burke was executed (and then dissected) in 1829 and Hare (who had testified against Burke) was released. Burke's skeleton and death mask are kept at

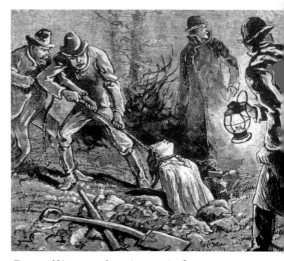

Grave-robbing was a lucrative practice for resurrectionists supplying medical schools

of the Flemish anatomist Andreas Vesalius (1514–63), who horrified the medical world by overturning the long-cherished teachings of Galen. He also changed the conventional method of teaching anatomy, in which the anatomist had lectured while a barber-surgeon carried out the dissection. Like Mondino dei' Luzzi (see p.23), Vesalius carried out his own dissections. He also introduced the use of detailed anatomical illustrations to show the interior structures of the body. This may seem like an obvious method now, but it was unprecedented at the time. In 1543, at the age of only 28, he published his work on the structure of the human body (*De humani corporis fabrica libri septem – On the fabric of the human body in seven books*) and raised a storm of outrage. He showed where Galen was wrong about the structure of the liver, the bile duct, the uterus, the upper jaw and the heart. In the case of the heart he demonstrated that blood does not pass from the right to the left ventricle by flowing

ANDREAS VESALIUS (1514–63)

Born in Flanders, Vesalius was the son of the court apothecary and the grandson of the physician to Emperor Maximilian. He took an interest in anatomy from an early age, dissecting the bodies of the dogs, cats and rats he found in the streets. After training at Louvain, Montpellier and Paris he moved to Padova (Padua) in Italy in 1537, where he was appointed professor of medicine and anatomy at the age of 23. So enthusiastic was he about his anatomical studies that when he came across a skeleton with its ligaments intact hanging on a gibbet near Louvain, he took it down and carried it home to investigate. Stealing bodies and skeletons from gibbets and charnel houses kept him supplied with specimens for his studies. He published his *Six Anatomical Tables (Tabulae anatomicae sex)* in 1538,

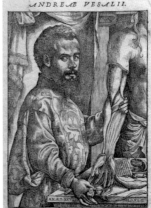

repeating the errors of Galen. When he produced his master work five years later, he corrected the mistakes Galen had made. Daring to challenge Galen brought the wrath of the medical establishment and the Catholic Church down on Vesalius's head. Reeling under the blows, he resigned his chair, burned all his unpublished works and became private physician to the Holy Roman Emperor Charles V and later to King Philip II of Spain. He died in a shipwreck on the island of Zakynthos on his way back from a trip to the Holy Land. Legend has it that the trip was a pilgrimage that had been demanded by the Inquisition in lieu of the death penalty, after he had dissected a Spanish nobleman whose heart was found to be still beating. Sadly, there is no evidence to support this exciting tale.

through invisible pores in the septum. He made it clear that Galen had based his human biology on the investigation of animals and that this had led to errors.

Vesalius revolutionized medicine. By popularizing dissection and creating detailed anatomical drawings he laid the foundations for modern anatomy. Using his methods, together with the experimental methods that were evolving in all areas of science, medical scientists around Europe began to unpick the body and finally discover how it really works.

William Harvey and the circulation of the blood

People have long recognized that blood is special. The Assyrians rightly supposed that blood was the life force of the body, but they thought that it collected in the liver, which was therefore the seat of life. In the 5th century BC the Pythagorean School taught that the heart was the centre of the circulatory system and that the breath of life, or *pneuma*, was taken in through the windpipe and carried around the body by the blood vessels.

Galen identified three connected systems in the body: the circulatory system, the respiratory system, and the digestive system. He also distinguished between arteries and veins, but he did not properly understand their function. His theory was that the heart sent life-giving energy or spirit through the arteries while the liver formed blood from food and fed it into the body through the veins. The blood did not circulate, he thought, but rather ebbed and flowed around the body in an undirected and rather desultory fashion. According to

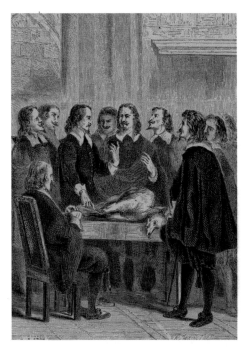

William Harvey studied the workings of the heart using dogs and other animals as subjects during controlled experiments

Galen's thinking, the blood eventually disappeared after being used up as nourishment by the tissues, some of it being converted to new flesh. It was then replaced by new blood from the liver. Galen believed that some blood leaked from the right to the left ventricle of the heart through invisibly small pores in the septum and there mixed with air. He also conjectured that a little of this blood was processed in nerves at the base of the skull and in the brain to make psychic *pneuma*, which conveys sensations. Despite his many errors, Galen made a significant breakthrough in demonstrating that the arteries contained only blood and not air as had previously been thought. He showed this by opening the artery of a dog under water in order to demonstrate that no bubbles rose from the poor animal's wound.

The 13th-century Arab scholar Ala al-Din Abu al-Hassan Ali ibn Abi-Hazm al-Qurashi al-Dimashqi (Ibn al-Nafis) pointed out some errors in Galen's model of the circulation. The heart had only two ventricles, not three, he said, and there were no pores in the septum. Ibn al-Nafis also stated that blood somehow mixes with air in the alveoli of the lungs and that the blood that leaves the heart through the pulmonary artery is the same as that which returns to the heart through the pulmonary vein. He anticipated the discovery of capillaries by stating that the pulmonary artery and the pulmonary vein must be connected in some way.

But Ibn al-Nafis' work had little impact and Galen's model of the heart and the circulation survived unchallenged in

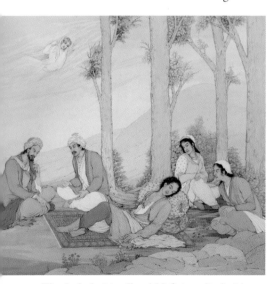

The Arab physician Ibn al-Nafis is credited with discovering the circulation of blood between the heart and lungs

Europe for almost 1,500 years. Speaking out against the Galenic model was considered heretical – literally. In 1553 the Spanish physician and theologian Michael Servetus suggested that the heart controlled the circulation of the blood and that the septum was not porous. He was burned at the stake for heresy in the same year, along with his books. (His model of the heart was not his only crime.) Galen had made many errors by basing human anatomy on that of animals, but Vesalius faced an outcry when he attempted to rectify the situation and he was forced to surrender his professorial chair as a consequence. In 1559, Italian anatomist Realdo Colombo presented evidence that supported the model of pulmonary circulation suggested by al-Nafis and Servetus, but it still had no significant impact.

It was the Englishman William Harvey (1578–1657) who finally unlocked the secret. Born in Folkestone, England, he studied under Hieronymus Fabricius at the University of Padova (Padua) while Galileo Galilei was teaching there. After Harvey had returned to England, he stated in 1603 that the blood moves constantly 'in a circular manner' and is driven by the action of the heart. Then in 1616 he gave lectures that built on Colombo's model. He suggested that the heart worked as a muscular pump, forcing the blood around the body. The heart did not, as previously believed, suck blood in and the blood vessels did not move the blood by themselves. Aerated blood, Harvey explained, is pushed from the left ventricle through the aorta to all parts of the body, travelling through ever smaller blood vessels on its journey.

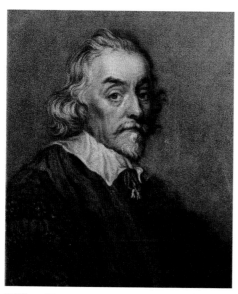

William Harvey was the first man in the western world to understand the circulation of the blood

Deaerated blood returns in the veins to the right atrium, and from there it is forced into the right ventricle and sent to the lungs by way of the pulmonary artery. There it is aerated, becoming arterial blood again. It then returns to the heart by entering the left atrium, and is moved by the systolic contraction of the heart into the left ventricle. The valves in the blood vessels, first described by Fabricius, prevent the blood from flowing backwards.

All that was missing was a demonstration of the existence of the capillaries and that was provided in 1661 by Marcello Malpighi. Since he did not use a microscope to look for the capillaries, Harvey was only able to theorize about the mechanism by which arterial blood that had been distributed to the extremities began its return journey as venous blood. He demonstrated that it must do so by using a

ligature to restrict the blood flow in an arm. The veins in the arm became swollen as they filled with blood. This proved that the blood that had flowed outwards through the arteries would have returned to the heart through the veins if the ligature had not been applied. It also showed that blood can only flow in one direction, as Fabricius had discovered.

THINGS INFINITESIMAL

The anatomists gradually discovered the real structure of the organs and tissues of the body and how they were related to each other. The new microscopes, first developed in the Netherlands in the late 16th century, enabled them to investigate ever smaller parts.

When Antonie van Leeuwenhoek (1632–1723) developed a microscope that could, for the first time, reveal micro-organisms and single cells, he did what any teenage boy would do and looked at his own sperm, blood and spit. Microscopes of lower power had been in use in the Netherlands since 1595 and Galileo had devised a compound microscope (with more than one lens), which he called the *occhiolino*, in 1625. But Leeuwenhoek's simple, single-lens microscope could magnify specimens up to 200 times – which was ten times more powerful than the early compound microscopes. Leeuwenhoek had no formal scientific education – in fact he worked as a draper – but he had endless curiosity and was very skilful at grinding lenses. The fineness of linen was judged by counting its threads, so Leeuwenhoek probably became familiar with magnifying lenses while he was working with cloth. He employed an

JOHN AUBREY, BRIEF LIVES – AN ACCOUNT OF WILLIAM HARVEY

Brief Lives is a treasure house of portraits of 16th-century figures, all drawn from life. Aubrey recalls that Harvey referred to Paracelsus as 'shitt-breeches' and wrote very poor Latin – his treatise on the circulation of the blood had to be translated for him by one Sir George Ent. He tells a chilling tale about Harvey travelling as a young man:

> *When Doctor Harvey (one of the Physitians College in London) being a Young Man, went to Travel towards Padoa: he went to Dover (with several others) and shewed his Pass, as the rest did, to the Governor there. The Governor told him, that he must not go, but he must keep him Prisoner. The Doctor desired to know for what reason? how he has transgrest. Well, it was his Will to have it so. The Pacquet Boat Hoisted Sail in the Evening (which was very clear) and the Doctor's Companions in it. There ensued a terrible Storme, and the Pacquet-Boat and all the Passengers were Drown'd: The next day the sad News was brought to Dover. The Doctor was unknown to the Governor, both by Name and Face; but the Night before, the Governor had a perfect Vision in a Dream of Doctor Harvey, who came to pass over to Calais; and that he had a Warning to stop him. This the Governor told to the Doctor the next day.*

Aubrey also related that Harvey had a quick and violent temper – 'this Dr. would be apt to draw-out his dagger upon every slight occasion' – that he drank coffee before it was fashionable to do so and that wherever he went he was inclined to go on excursions into the woods to look for interesting natural things 'so that my Lord Ambassador [in Vienna] would be really angry with him, for there was not only the danger of Thieves, but also of wild beasts'. He also reported that Harvey's practice declined after he published his work on the circulation, because people thought him 'crack-brained'. But not all was bad, Aubrey went on, because, according to Hobbes, 'he is the only man, perhaps, that ever lived to see his owne Doctrine established in his life-time'.

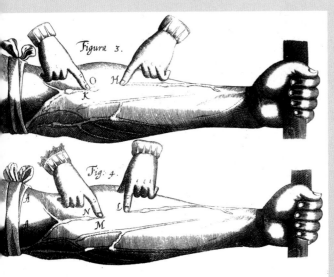

Harvey's demonstration of the blood flow in the arm

BLOOD TRANSFUSIONS

The specialness of blood has led to many strange notions about its power. Some psychopaths have believed that drinking it or bathing in it would give them eternal youth or potency; and some physicians have hoped to save lives by either removing it from their patients or adding more. The earliest attempts at blood transfusions used the blood of animals, with unfortunate results. Jean-Baptiste Denis, physician to Louis XIV of France, first tried a transfusion in the winter of 1667. His subject was a madman who had taken to wandering the streets of Paris naked, generally after beating his wife and before setting fire to houses. Denis drained ten ounces of blood from the man and then attached a tube to a calf's artery. He hoped that the calf's tranquillity would be transferred to the patient along with the blood. After several transfusions, the poor madman became very ill and Denis stopped. The patient remained stable for a while, with no more wife-beating or house-burning excursions, so Denis claimed success for his treatment. It did not end well, though – the patient's wife tried to persuade Denis to repeat the treatment, which he refused to do. Shortly afterwards, the woman administered a fatal dose of arsenic to her husband. The bad publicity led to a ban on transfusions, first in France and then in Great Britain. A similar ban was then imposed by the pope.

Successful blood transfusions between humans were not possible until the early 20th century, when the Austrian Karl Landsteiner discovered and categorized human blood groups A, B, O, and AB. Armed with this knowledge, Landsteiner showed that transfusions between humans with compatible blood types did not lead to the clumping and destruction of cells observed by Leonard Landois in 1875 when he gave patients transfusions from animals or randomly selected human donors.

Karl Landsteiner received the Nobel Prize for his discovery of blood groups

illustrator to draw what he could see through his microscope and he wrote detailed descriptions of his observations. He was the first man to see bacteria. In 1683 he wrote a letter to the Royal Society in London describing what he had seen in the plaque taken from an old man who had never cleaned his teeth: '... an unbelievably great company of living animalcules, a-swimming more nimbly than any I had ever seen up to this time'. Initial resistance to his 'animalcules' was quelled when the respected figure Robert Hooke confirmed his findings.

LEEUWENHOEK'S SAMPLES REVISITED

A collection of letters and samples prepared by Leeuwenhoek and sent to the Royal Society in London was discovered in the archives in 1981, 300 years after he sent them. He had prepared his samples in a way similar to modern methods and with such care and skill that they can still be viewed and yield good results today. By recreating a single-lens microscope the same as that which Leeuwenhoek used it has been possible to see exactly what he saw, and even identify the mites that he caught in his house, magnified to 200 times their actual size.

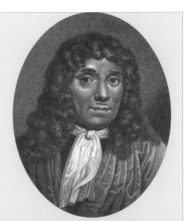

Antoine van Leeuwenhoek – the first man to see bacteria

Marcello Malpighi, who discovered the blood capillaries, examined tissues from the liver, the spleen, the lungs, the skin, the brain and various glands. The microscope soon revealed red blood cells, too. Robert Hooke was the first person to observe that plant tissue is made up of cells. When he published his famous *Micrographia* in 1665, which reproduced what he had seen through the lens of the microscope, the English diarist Samuel Pepys described it as 'the most ingenious book that I ever read in my life'.

Improved microscopes in the 18th century allowed the anatomists to look ever

Marie-François-Xavier Bichat

more closely, exploring the workings of the human body still further. Marie-François-Xavier Bichat (1771–1802) described 21 different types of tissue, present in several organs that perform different functions. He maintained that diseases should be considered as problems with particular tissues rather than whole organs. Zooming in even more closely, in 1839 Theodor Schwann was the first to discover that human and animal bodies are made up of cells similar to the plant cells identified by Robert Hooke. He identified different types of cells and looked at their structure, thereby establishing the field of cytology. But it was Rudolf Virchow (1821–1902), a German professor of anatomy, who showed how cells are at the heart of all biological activity including growth and

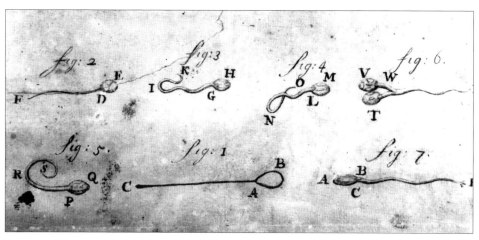

Leeuwenhoek's drawings of his own sperm – the first ever seen

reproduction. He also realized that cancer is the result of abnormal cells running out of control and multiplying furiously.

A mechanistic model

As dissection revealed the large structures inside the body and the microscope revealed the different organs, tissues and cells that made it up, a different type of intellectual model of the body became possible. Scientists considered the body in a new light, trying to make sense of the structures that the anatomists had revealed. Newton's demonstrations of optics elucidated the working of the eye, Galileo Galilei's search for mathematical laws governing all phenomena showed muscles and bones working as levers, and Santorio Santorio (or Sanctorius) applied physics and chemistry to the human body in the first studies of the metabolism. Scientists began to see the body as a collection of mechanical processes. The healthy body, like a

well-oiled machine, would run itself with minimal attention as long as it was provided with suitable fuel and working conditions. Illness was a spanner in the works. Herman Boerhaave (1668–1738) adopted a mechanical, hydraulic model – he saw the body as a system of balanced pressures and flows of bodily fluids. For the philosopher René Descartes (1596–1650), the body was a machine that ran like clockwork.

In 1670, John Mayow showed that air is drawn into the lungs by enlarging the thoracic cavity. He demonstrated this principle by using a pair of bellows, inside which was a bladder. When the bellows were expanded the bladder filled with air. Although he could not explain the exchange of gases in the blood, with oxygen being absorbed and carbon dioxide released, he had established the mechanical principle of respiration. Bellows became the basic tool of artificial

Leeuwenhoek's microscope

33

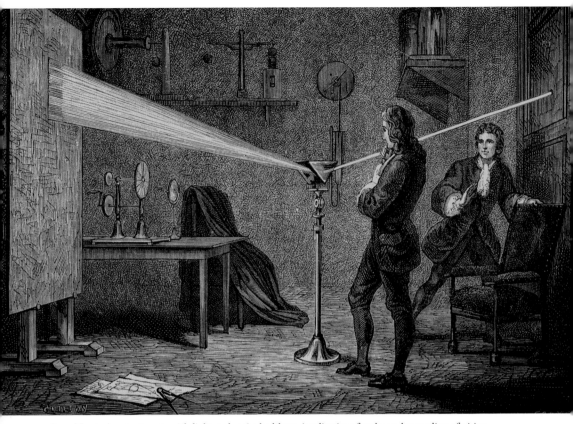

Isaac Newton's experiments with light and optics had huge implications for the understanding of vision

respiration, which was first explored in the late 18th century when doctors became interested in resuscitating people who had nearly died. More complex mechanical respirators were unsuccessful until 1889, when an American doctor, O.W. Doe, produced a box respirator to resuscitate stillborn infants. After placing the child inside, with only the mouth and the nose exposed, the operator intermittently blew through a pipe to push air into the box, increasing the pressure. When the pressure was released, air was pulled into the child's lungs through the nose and the mouth.

Chemical reactions

The model of the body as a mechanical system was soon challenged by the emerging science of chemistry. The French chemist Antoine Lavoisier (1743–94) made the first breakthrough by describing the chemical process of respiration as one in which the body takes in oxygen and exhales carbon dioxide. As such, he showed that oxygen was essential to life, likening the process to combustion. The German chemist Justus von Liebig (1803–73) saw the body as a whole collection of chemical systems that controlled all aspects of the

SANTORIO SANTORIO (SANCTORIUS) (1561–1636)

Santorio graduated from the University of Padova in 1582 and later returned as its Professor of Theoretical Medicine from 1611 to 1624. He carried out an extraordinary experiment in which he spent a period of 30 years constantly weighing himself, the food and drink he took in, and the waste matter he produced. Much of his time was spent in a weighing chair he devised for the purpose. Santorio found that the mass of his excrement and urine was much smaller than the mass of the food and drink he had consumed, so he came up with a theory of 'insensible perspiration' to account for the difference. His attempt to use mathematics to try to understand the workings of the body was a breakthrough, and it established the model of the body as a machine. In addition to his experiments with weight, Santorio produced a graded thermometer and a meter for measuring the pulse rate, called a 'pulsilogium'. It is likely, though, that others working in Venice at the same time contributed to these developments.

metabolism. He explained the workings of respiration, the release of energy, and the production of waste. By measuring what went into the body and what came out, and analysing body fluids, he established the field of biochemistry.

A MAGICAL TRANSFORMATION?

Those who favoured a mechanistic model were often in conflict with those who favoured a model founded in chemistry. The digestive system was a hotly contested battleground, for both mechanics and chemistry play a part.

The means by which the body processes food into flesh and blood (and waste) had puzzled medical scientists from the time of Aristotle. The Hippocratic philosophers believed that food was first reduced to a liquid form by heat, after which it was converted into the four humours and absorbed into the body. Two hundred years later, the more enlightened Erasistratus suggested that digestion is primarily a mechanical process. He explained the activity we can feel after eating as the action of muscles churning and squashing food to break it up. However, Galen dismissed Erasistratus' ideas, stating that nutritious material was carried to the liver and made into blood through the action of heat. Such was Galen's standing that the heat theory went unchallenged again for nearly 1,500 years.

CHEMICAL SOUP AND MUSCLE MACHINERY

The Dutch physician Franz De Le Boë, or Franciscus Sylvius (1614–72), suggested that digestion was a chemical process. He studied gastric juices and saliva and concluded that digestion was like fermentation. In the other camp, the Italian mathematician Giovanni Borelli (1608–79)

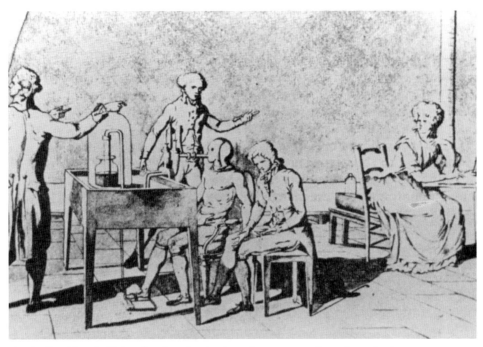

Antoine Lavoisier, the 'father of modern chemistry', carries out an experiment in respiration

likened the stomach to a machine that grinds food into tiny particles. The pendulum swung in favour of chemistry in 1752, with the work of the French physiologist René de Réaumur (1683–1757). Réaumur fed a hawk two metal tubes stuffed with meat and covered at the ends with gauze. The hawk eventually regurgitated the tubes, but the meat had been digested – dissolved, Réaumur concluded, by gastric juices, since muscular activity could not have reached inside the protective tubes.

The Italian biologist Lazzaro Spallanzani (1729–99) repeated Réaumur's experiments with his own hawks, but he went even further. Evidently not a squeamish man, he began by immersing minced meat in tubes of gastric juice which

he then incubated in his armpits for three days at a time. Encouraged by the results, he examined the process in situ by swallowing items attached to a thread and leaving them in his stomach for a while, before withdrawing them by pulling on the thread. He proved conclusively that food is dissolved by the actions of chemicals – though he did not identify the mix of stomach acid and enzymes that was involved. That remained for William Beaumont to study.

A WINDOW INTO THE STOMACH

While stationed near Michigan in 1822, army surgeon William Beaumont (1785–1853) was called upon to treat Alexis St Martin, a French-Canadian trapper who had been shot accidentally at

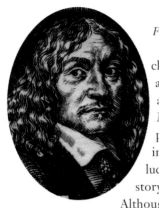

Franciscus Sylvius

close range. It was an unfortunate accident for St Martin – he lost part of his abdominal wall – but a lucky break for the story of medicine. Although St Martin's injury healed, it never sealed up completely, and he was left with a hole through which the resourceful Beaumont carried out more than 200 experiments over a period of nine

years. Beaumont fed St Martin a variety of foods and timed their digestion. He discovered that vegetables were the least digestible food while milk coagulates before it is digested. He collected gastric juice and sent it for chemical analysis. This revealed the presence of hydrochloric acid, which conclusively established the role of chemistry in digestion.

THE GHOST IN THE MACHINE

If the body was a composite of physical, mechanical and chemical systems that could be explained by science, one important question remained unanswered

LAZZARO SPALLANZANI (1729–99)

Spallanzani started to study law at the University of Bologna, but the famous natural philosopher and mathematician Laura Bassi (also his cousin) swayed him towards science. His interests and his expertise were wide. He disproved the theory of spontaneous generation and demonstrated – before Louis Pasteur was born – that micro-organisms in liquid can be killed by boiling and do not reappear if the container is sealed. He performed the first artificial insemination (of a dog), explained the physics of skipping stones over the surface of a pond, successfully transplanted the heads of snails, investigated the echo location methods used by bats and laid the foundations of modern vulcanology and meteorology.

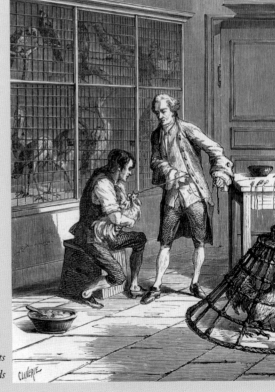

Spallanzani carrying out his experiments in digestion on birds

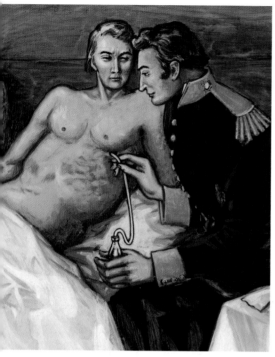

William Beaumont took samples of partly digested food from his patient over a period of nine years and established the role of chemistry in human digestion

– what made it a living, thinking, conscious being? There were three approaches to this question in 17th-century Europe. The animists believed that the immortal soul animated the body, and that put an end to their enquiries. With the exception of René Descartes, who proclaimed with confidence that the soul resided in the pineal gland, scientists were unwilling to locate the soul. Georg Stahl went as far as to say, in 1708, that the body putrefies when the soul leaves it and that illness is the soul's attempt to rid the body of morbid matter – but that the nature of the soul must remain unknown and unknowable.

Two other schools of thought, vitalism and mechanism, provided more of a platform for discussion. Vitalists felt that some form of vital spirit or force animated the body and distinguished living from non-living matter. The mechanist view was that the body could be fully explained by science – by the mechanism of the muscles and the organs and, later, the chemistry of body processes.

VITAL SPIRITS

In the mid 18th century, Albrecht von Haller (1708–1777) demonstrated the differences between muscle and nerve fibre, laying the foundations of neurophysiology. Haller used the 'irritability' of muscle fibre and the 'sensitivity' of nerve fibre to explain how the heart pumped blood, something William Harvey had been unable to account for. This difference in the fibres, to Haller's mind, showed that the body was animated by a vital force that was beyond the scope of science. But scientists still remained keen to investigate it. Candidates for the vital spirit included 'vital heat', oxygen and, later, electricity (explored by Galvani and Volta). The Scot John Brown suggested that all fibres were 'excitable' – life was generated by constant stimulus; illness resulted if there was too much or too little stimulus. This led him to a simple treatment regime which was based on administering either a stimulant or depressant – laudanum or whisky – in all cases. The simplicity of the system made it popular, but Brown died of alcohol abuse at the age of 53, making its efficacy suspect.

In 1751 Robert Whytt suggested that an 'unconscious sentient principle' activated the nerves. Then in the mid 1780s the Italian Luigi Galvani showed, by an experiment that involved hanging frogs' legs from copper wires on an iron balcony, that electricity would make muscles twitch. When electricity was used to revive a child who had apparently died after falling from a window in 1788 – the first attempt at defibrillation – the case for electricity as the vital force was strengthened for those inclined to believe it.

The idea of vitalism was first challenged experimentally in 1828, when Freidrich Wöhler (1800–82) managed to create the organic material urea from ammonia and cyanogen. In order to excuse the embarrassing implications of the discovery, Wöhler suggested that some residual vital spirit had survived from the animal source of his ingredients. Experiments conducted directly with animals also suggested that there was nothing very special about living tissue. Réaumur – who fed his hawk tubes of meat (see p.36) – showed that lobsters could regrow claws they had lost. Then in 1744 Abraham Trembley demonstrated that fresh-water hydra could be split, generating entirely new individuals. Proof that no vital spirit is needed for the activity of an organism came in 1897 when Eduard Buchner showed that an extract of ground-up yeast cells could still produce fermentation even though

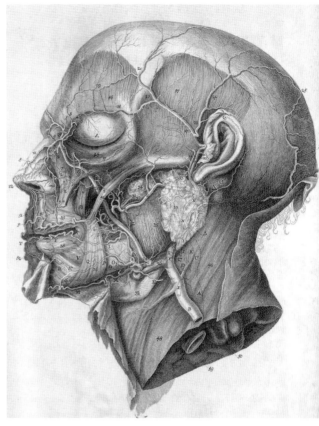

The human head as Albrecht von Haller saw it

Albrecht von Haller

there were no cells present. The effect was correctly identified as the result of enzymes, which had been named by Wilhelm Kühne in 1876.

The brain in control

If there is any place in which some vital spirit or soul resides, the brain is a good candidate. Herophilos considered the brain to be the command centre of the body and the seat of intelligence; the ancient

Egyptians noticed that damage to the brain or the spinal cord could result in physical disability; and Galen correctly identified the brain and the nerves as being responsible for sensation and thought. Confirmation that the brain is also the source of personality came after Phineas Gage's terrible accident on the American railroads in 1848 (see opposite).

Attempts to map physical functions to different areas of the brain began with the ancient Greeks, who believed that there was an area where 'vital spirit' became 'animal spirit' and was then sent out into the rest of the body. In the European Middle Ages, three functions were identified – imagination, memory and intelligence – together with the corresponding areas of the brain.

Although some medical writers tried to ascribe physical and sensory functions to particular areas of the brain, real progress could only be made by examining the effects of illness and brain injury, such as that suffered by Phineas Gage. This often depended on post-mortem examination, when damaged areas could be related to loss of function, but there were exceptions. Roger Sperry (1913–94) and Michael Gazzaniga (b.1939) experimented on people whose corpus callosum (the connection between the two halves of the brain) had been severed, usually as a treatment for extreme epilepsy. They found that each half of the brain is responsible for

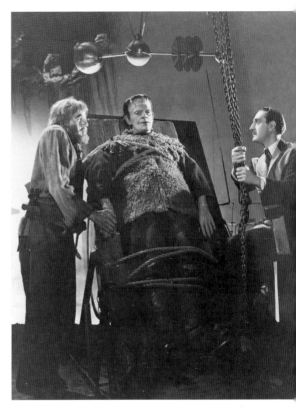

Electricity was the 'vital spirit' animating Frankenstein's monster

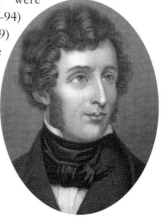
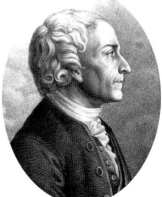

Friedrich Wöhler (left) and Abraham Trembley (right)

PHINEAS GAGE'S ACCIDENT

In 1848 Phineas Gage was working as the foreman of a gang constructing railways when a freak accident blew a three-foot-long iron rod straight through his head. It entered through his cheek bone and left through the crown. Astonishingly, Gage made a complete physical recovery, but he was a changed person. He had been sociable and easygoing before the accident, but afterwards he became bad-tempered and foul-mouthed, impossible to live or work with and given to snap decisions – often foolish ones. It became clear that some aspects of personality and thought depended on the physical brain. Gage ended up as an exhibit in P.T. Barnum's museum of freaks until he died of a seizure at the age of 38.

Nearly 150 years after Gage's death his body, together with the rod that had been buried with him, was exhumed. A computer reconstruction of the accident revealed the parts of Gage's brain that had been destroyed by the accident. This indicated where the functions of decision-making and social awareness take place.

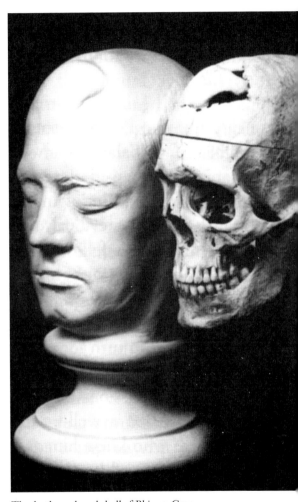

The death mask and skull of Phineas Gage

Tell me where is fancy bred,
Or in the heart or in the head,
How begot, how nourished?
        The Merchant of Venice (William
            Shakespeare), Act III, Scene ii

particular types of mental activity. For example, if there is no connection between the two halves of the brain a person may know the word for something but might not be able to say what the thing is for. In 1981 Sperry won a Nobel Prize for his

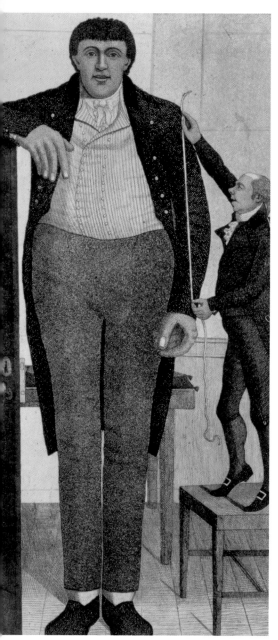

The 'Irish Giant', Charles O'Brien, was 8ft 4in tall. He paid fishermen £500 to dump his body at sea to prevent dissection after his death (1783), but a doctor made a counter-bid and won his skeleton

work on brain function. The advent of MRI and CAT scanning has now made it possible to observe the workings of the brain. A trace chemical (usually a radioactive sugar) is introduced, and this shows up on the scan, revealing which areas of the brain are used as the subject carries out different types of mental activity.

THE ILLUSORY IMAGE OF PERFECTION

We have seen how the models of the body have evolved over time, but have so far concentrated on the normal healthy body. Before turning to models of disease it is worth pausing to consider how the sick, the disfigured or the different body has been viewed. The body that has been afflicted by sickness, broken by injury or differently moulded through disability or deformity has been variously seen as an abomination, an object of pity – something to be hidden or corrected – or as a wonder. In ancient Sparta, disabled children were exposed on a mountainside to die, but the Aztecs had a goddess with special responsibility for deformed children, Atlatonan. The Olmecs of pre-Columbian South America appear to have thought that children with Down's syndrome were the product of copulation with a jaguar, which made them were-jaguars.

Birth deformities have sometimes been seen as a sign of the mother's infidelity, or as divine punishment for some crime or sin committed by one of the parents, or even an ancestor. At other times, the opposite view has prevailed. Writing in the mid 16th century, when intolerance was more common than inclusiveness, Michel de Montaigne wrote:

Those which we call monsters are not so with God, who in the immensitie of his worke seeth the infinitie of formes therein contained.

Depictions of congenital deformity often appeared in collections of wonders, alongside such unlikely creatures as unicorns and giraffes. They were often accompanied by scientific explanations. One such book was *On Monsters and Marvels*, an examination of human and animal birth defects and their likely causes, written by Ambroise Paré, the famous surgeon. From conjoined twins to individuals with missing or extra limbs, Paré accounts for abnormalities by citing such causes as the glory or the wrath of God; too much or too little 'seed' (semen); corrupt seed; mingled seed (because a woman has had intercourse with two men); misbehaviour of the mother; damage to the mother; the mother's imagination; too narrow a womb; and the influence of demons or devils.

In some places, birth defects are still seen as either a blessing or a curse. To medical eyes, a girl born in India in 2005 with four arms and four legs was a conjoined twin, though her twin had no independent torso or head. But many people in India saw her as a reincarnation of the goddess Lakshmi. When an operation to separate her from her 'spare'

WHAT ARE WE REALLY LIKE?

Whatever the generally accepted model of the human body, people have very different perceptions of their own body. When there is a mismatch between our image of ourselves and the way others see us, it could be an indication of mental illness. People with anorexia often think they look fat, even if to others they are skeletally thin. But there are far more bizarre forms of misperception. Cotard's syndrome sufferers believe themselves to be dead – walking corpses. Someone with Alice in Wonderland syndrome may feel that they are very tiny, or very large, or extremely wide. Lycanthropes believe themselves to be werewolves, or feel that they look like wolves. An individual who suffers from Koro believes that his genitals are shrinking into his body.

arms and legs was carried out in 2007, western science hailed it as a wonderful act that had given the girl the chance of a normal life. But some of her Indian neighbours felt that it was a violation of a miraculous being.

By branding physically different people as monsters, or even wonders, people who see themselves as normal are creating a closed club. Their 'us' and 'them' mentality gives them licence to treat 'them' badly. At its worst, this polarity of sick and well, different and 'normal', can lead to the practice of eugenics – the restriction of the gene pool and the 'purging' of people who are considered inferior. Some people express concern that modern prenatal screening and the selection of embryos for IVF (in vitro fertilization) are resurrecting the spectre of eugenics and attempting to eliminate conditions such as Down's syndrome and

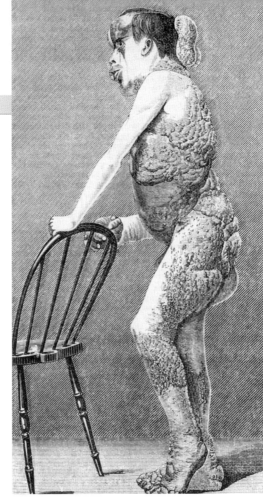

THE ELEPHANT MAN

John Merrick was born in Leicestershire in 1862. By the time he was three years old bumps had started to appear on the left side of his body. He eventually became so severely disfigured and disabled that he was forced to make a living by exhibiting himself as a freak. In 1886 he was taken into the care of the physician Frederick Treves, and moved into the London Hospital as a permanent resident. Merrick became a celebrity in London society and developed a wide circle of friends, but he was still subjected to staring and abuse from people he did not know. He died in his sleep at the age of 27, as a result of his condition.

John Merrick showing the alarming extent of his deformity

autism, as well as other non-fatal conditions which affect quality of life.

For the first time in history we have the power to model the bodies of the future according to a generally accepted idea of normality or perfection. It is a power that could easily be abused, so costing us the richness and diversity of humanity. But at the same time it is a power that could save future generations from debilitating conditions and disabilities. Whether we put this power to good use or lay it aside is a decision that will take careful consideration and negotiation.

THE BODY POLITIC

It has often been impossible for medical scientists to call the prevailing model of the body into question because it has been upheld by a ruling elite, religious belief or simply the tyranny of tradition. Judaeo-Christian tradition holds that the body is created in the image of God, but that humankind is fallen. The concept of the fallen nature of humanity explains why the flesh is subject to so many ills, but at the same time it nurtures the idea that the healthy body is the image of perfection. It is a belief that has also, at some times, made the body

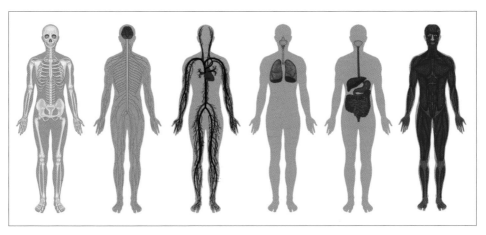

Modern-day western medicine divides the human body into separate systems

inviolate – a notion that has restricted medical progress in many cultures. Without the ability to examine the body, through dissection and microscopic observation, it is impossible to come to an informed, scientific understanding of how it works. Medical systems that do not encourage or allow such physical examination remain stuck with a model that is not able to take advantage of the advances of modern science.

Modern medical science in the West divides the body into systems by function: the respiratory system, the digestive system, the circulatory system, the musculo-skeletal system and the nervous system. These systems comprise organs, tissues and cells and their operation involves chemical and physical processes. Our current (still incomplete) understanding of the working of the human body is the product of more than 2,500 years' investigation, exploration and experimentation. The medical models which have not allowed investigation have remained pretty much where they were

2,000 years ago. There has developed a dichotomy between the holistic or spiritually-based medical philosophies of the East, rooted in traditional beliefs, and the medicine of the West, founded on scientific method and investigation. It remains to be seen whether systems that appear to have developed into polar opposites can be usefully brought together in the future.

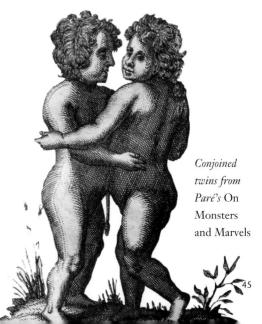

Conjoined twins from Paré's On Monsters and Marvels

45

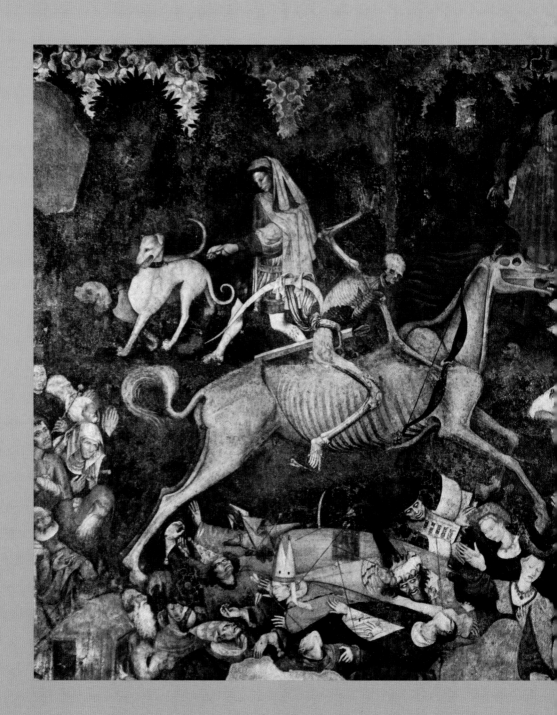

CHAPTER 2

MODELS OF DISEASE

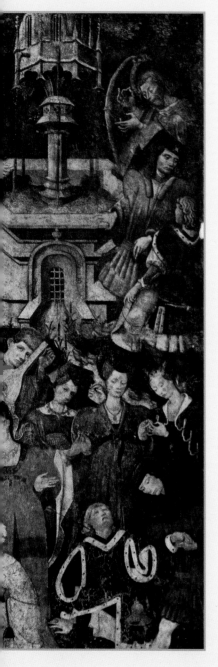

Our response to a disease is governed by our understanding of its nature and its causes. Our earliest ancestors imagined that diseases were created by mysterious and invisible forces, such as evil spirits, vengeful gods, curses or the malign influence of the stars. The dawning of scientific thought led people to look for more immediate causes – imbalances of humours, blocked energies or oozing, evil miasmas became the culprits. Then 400 years ago the microscope added previously invisible organisms to the list of possibilities. But although they could be seen, these micro-organisms were not positively linked to contagion until the 19th century. At last, the role of bacteria, viruses and parasites came to light. Meanwhile, the study of chemistry and physiology revealed other culprits. The workings of the body itself, the environment and our own behaviour can all be the source of illness. Vitamins, hormones, enzymes and various toxins all have their parts to play in health and sickness. The world may still seem to hold danger and disease lurking around every corner, just as it did for our ancestors, even though we account for it differently.

Death, in the form of plague, rode roughshod over the populations of Europe and Asia in the 14th century, cutting down rich and poor alike

ALL MANNER OF SICKNESS

In John Milton's *Paradise Lost*, Adam is shown the consequences of the Fall, including the illnesses that will beset mankind. The following excerpt provides an illuminating catalogue of the conditions that were recognized and feared in the 17th century.

Immediately a place
Before his eyes appeared, sad, noisome, dark;
A lazar-house it seemed, wherein were laid
Numbers of all diseased; all maladies
Of ghastly spasm, or racking torture, qualms
Of heart-sick agony, all feverous kinds,
Convulsions, epilepsies, fierce catarrhs,
Intestine stone and ulcer, colic pangs,
Demoniac frenzy, moping melancholy,
And moon-struck madness, pining atrophy,
Marasmus, and wide-wasting pestilence,
Dropsies, and asthmas, and joint-racking
rheums.
Dire was the tossing, deep the groans.
Despair tended the sick; busiest from couch
to couch;
And over them triumphant Death his dart
Shook, but delayed to strike, though oft invoked
With vows, as their chief good, and final hope.

Book XI, 477–93

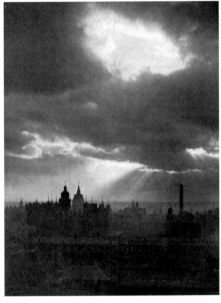

By the 17th century, crowded cities such as Edinburgh were hotbeds of sickness and disease

Supernatural agency

Disease often seems to spring from nowhere, even today, but our ancestors would have found its causes or sources hard to imagine and impossible to see. For millennia, the very idea that illness could be caused by an invisibly small organism invading the body would have seemed bizarre and incredible. Instead, people were often inclined to believe that they had been cursed by a god or invaded by an evil spirit.

TOUCHED BY THE GODS?

We have no record of the medical beliefs of prehistoric humanity, but it seems likely that people believed evil spirits or angry gods visited disease upon them. Evidence from later societies certainly corroborates that view. The Edwin Smith papyrus (c.1600BC) refers to 'something entering from the outside', which causes disease, and goes on to explain that this may be the 'breath of a god'. About 3,000 years ago the Avesta, the holy book of the ancient Persian

Zoroastrians, described medicine as a fight against demons.

Following the practices laid down by religious authorities has sometimes had a genuine impact on health, even when that was not the intention of believers. Many of the rules laid down in the Book of Leviticus do indeed make a good hygiene code because they reduce the chances of food poisoning and infection. Unless seafood is very fresh, eating it in a hot country could easily lead to food poisoning; a divine pronouncement prohibiting it usefully saves believers from taking the risk. In ancient India, too, hygiene rules were an important part of the Hindu religion and they doubtless helped to keep followers healthy.

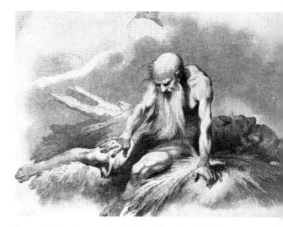

A vengeful god seemed a likely explanation for the mysterious arrival of sickness

Even when an immediate physical cause of sickness was visible, such as an infected wound or a parasite, people still believed that the hand of God was involved. This could lead to a fatalistic approach. Muslims and Christians alike have believed that it was the will of Allah or God that they were sick and that they would recover or die as the deity saw fit. This is not, of course, an attitude that leads to a rigorous search for a cure.

THE SACRED DISEASE

Some diseases have been particularly associated with the hand of God. The interpretation has often been ambivalent, particularly in the Judaeo-Christian tradition – was the sufferer blessed or cursed?

Ancient Indian texts and the Babylonian clay tablets gave recognizable accounts of many types of epileptic seizure, but both sources considered them to be associated with evil spirits of some sort, so they advised spiritual rather than physical

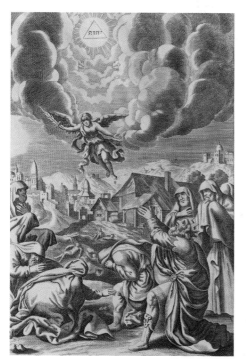

Divine retribution: God sends a plague as a punishment

treatment. A Babylonian description of epilepsy from c.650BC shows that a demon was considered responsible for the condition:

If at the time of his possession his mind is awake, the demon can be driven out; if at the time of his possession his mind is not so aware, the demon cannot be driven out.

Hippocrates was perhaps the first person to refute the idea that 'the sacred disease', as epilepsy was called, was the result of demonic possession or a visitation of the gods.

It is thus with regard to the disease called Sacred: it appears to me to be nowise more divine nor more sacred than other diseases, but has a natural cause like other affections.

But he could not identify the 'natural cause' so his words were of little help and general

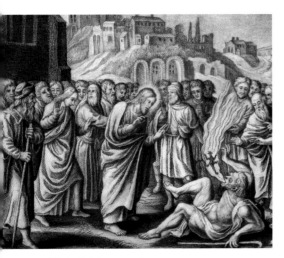

Christ driving out a demon

opinion remained unchanged. The Gospel of St Mark, written at least 500 years after Hippocrates, reports that Christ drove out a spirit from a young man. The spirit was said to have produced attacks in which the man, foaming at the mouth and unable to speak, became rigid and fell to the ground, gnashing his teeth – the classic symptoms of an epileptic seizure.

Often, sufferers were stigmatized, ostracized and punished. During the witch hunts of the later Middle Ages and the early Renaissance, seizures were taken as a sign of witchcraft, or of possession by a demon: countless innocent epileptics were doubtless executed for witchcraft. On the other hand, modern historians have suggested that some religious mystics were epileptic, so what appeared to be divinely-induced frenzies were perhaps no more than epileptic seizures. These more fortunate individuals were often revered – but sometimes they were derided as shams or heretics. Epilepsy was finally recognized as a neurological disorder after the British neurologist John Hughlings Jackson suggested in 1873 that seizures were caused by sudden, brief electrochemical discharges in the brain.

DISEASE AS A MORAL MEASURE

Leprosy, the scourge of the early Middle Ages, was frequently given a divine aspect by Christian writers. Guy de Chauliac (c.1300–68) wrote that leprosy was sent as a punishment from God. But he also claimed that lepers were enduring purgatory on earth and that their salvation was assured. Lepers in medieval Europe certainly had to endure a great deal – cast out of society

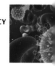

to live in leper colonies or lazar-houses, they were denied normal interaction with others and were stripped of their legal and civic status.

Leprosy was not the only disease that the gods might mete out to evil-doers. Syphilis – an alarming, new disease to 15th-century Europe – was often considered a mark of God's vengeance. The returning conquistadors and explorers brought the

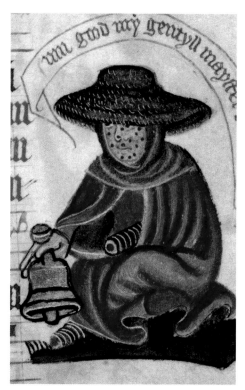

Medieval lepers had to carry a bell to warn others of their affliction and were ostracized from society through the inception of leper colonies

---

THE TESTAMENT OF CRESSEID

The Scots poet Robert Henryson wrote a continuation of Chaucer's Troilus and Criseyde in which the faithless Cresseid (Criseyde) is punished with leprosy by the gods. Because the setting is classical Greece, this time it is the Greek gods that are responsible.

Fra heit [heat] of bodie I the now depryve,
And to thy seiknes [sickness] sall be na recure [cure]
Bot in dolour [pain] thy dayis to indure.
Thy cristall ene mingit [eyes mingled] with blude I mak,
Thy voice sa cleir unplesand, hoir, and hace [unpleasant, rough and hoarse],
Thy lustie lyre [fair complexion] ovirspred with spottis blak,
And lumpis haw appeirand in thy face:
Quhair thow cummis, ilk man sall fle the place.
This [thus] sall thow go begging fra hous to hous
With cop [cup] and clapper [bell] lyke ane lazarous [leper].

---

disease to Europe from South America. It was a good swap for the smallpox, flu and measles that the Europeans had taken with them to the New World and which killed up to 90 per cent of the local population. European diseases raged through the New World, slaying far more people than the swords of the conquerors could ever have dispatched.

At that time, syphilis was considered to be God's revenge on the lustful and the promiscuous, since it was quite clearly related to sexual activity. Those of a scientific bent also recognized that syphilis

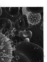

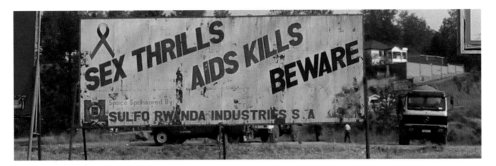

is sexually transmitted. An allegorical poem written in 1530 by the Italian physician Girolamo Fracastoro (c.1478–1553) has the shepherd Syphilis offend the sun god by worshipping another deity. The shepherd was afflicted with the disease as a punishment. Fracastoro gave the disease its name and wrote the first rigorous account of it.

In recent years, some people have adopted a similarly judgmental approach to AIDS. When the disease first emerged amongst the gay communities of the United

Rwanda, like much of sub-Saharan Africa, struggles to combat the AIDS epidemic. Education is a key tool to help raise awareness of the risks

States and Europe, some straight-laced moralists considered it a 'gay plague' sent by God – a vengeance directed against 'immoral' homosexual men. And some people believe that we should not seek or publicize cures for sexually transmitted diseases because they fear that doing so may encourage licentiousness. The threat of illness is seen by some as a useful

THE ROMANTIC DISEASE

In the 19th century, tuberculosis (TB) had a romantic image. Whereas many diseases produce ugly changes in the body, TB produces weight loss, an appealing pale skin and rosy cheeks. Writers made use of it to produce beautiful tragic heroes and heroines who faded away inexorably while retaining an ethereal beauty. TB was also thought to produce increased sexual energy and passion, particularly in women, which added to the erotic appeal of the heroines. The discomfort and pain that comes with the disease was glossed over.

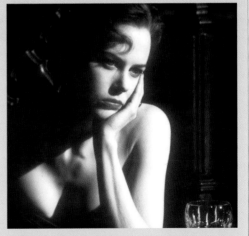

In Moulin Rouge, *the heroine's tubercular beauty is tragically alluring*

THREE-FOLD PLAGUE

The bacterium *Yersinia pestis* causes three types of plague:

Bubonic plague follows the bite of an infected flea, which introduces plague bacilli into the lymphatic system. This form of plague is characterized by horrifically painful buboes, which are swellings of the lymph nodes. Without modern antibiotic treatment around 60 per cent of victims will die in a few days.

Septicaemic plague is also caused by flea bites, but it occurs when the bacilli enter the bloodstream instead of the lymphatic system. Untreated, it is nearly always fatal within about 24 hours.

Pneumonic plague is caused by inhaling the bacillus in droplets that have been coughed or spat out by other plague victims. It is in this form that plague passes from person to person; it is highly contagious and usually fatal.

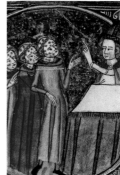

All three forms produce dark colouration in the skin, which is caused by subcutaneous bleeding (hence the name Black Death). Despite considerable differences in presentation, Guy de Chauliac recognized that bubonic and pneumonic plague were forms of the same disease and distinguished between them in his *Chirurgia magna* (1363).

Medieval plague victims receive guidance and comfort from a priest

---

way of policing morals, even in the 21st century.

WHOLESALE VENGEANCE

God could take revenge on a whole society, or even the whole world, as easily as He could wreak vengeance on a particular group or individual. After floods, plagues were considered the divine weapon of choice. The Old Testament speaks of the plagues of Egypt, which were sent directly by God as a punishment. They included a plague of boils and a plague of swellings in the private parts (usually translated as haemorrhoids), which may have been buboes in the groin.

The first certain account of bubonic plague described the Plague of Justinian which struck Europe in AD541–2, during the reign of the Byzantine emperor Justinian. Coming from Egypt to Constantinople (now Istanbul) it swept through the city, killing up to 10,000 people a day at its height – the dead lay unburied in the streets, according to the contemporary chronicler Procopius. By AD600 the plague had killed around 50 per cent of the population of Europe. It has been blamed for the onset of the so-called Dark Ages, when intellectual and cultural advances in Europe apparently came to a standstill for several centuries. When the physicians were unable to contain

PROCOPIUS ON THE PLAGUE OF JUSTINIAN

During these times there was a pestilence, by which the whole human race came near to being annihilated... it is quite impossible either to express in words or to conceive in thought any explanation, except indeed to refer it to God. For it did not come in a part of the world nor upon certain men, nor did it confine itself to any season of the year, so that from such circumstances it might be possible to find subtle explanations of a cause, but it embraced the entire world, and blighted the lives of all men... For it left [untouched] neither island nor cave nor mountain ridge which had human inhabitants...

... I am unable to say whether the cause of this diversity of symptoms was to be found in the difference in bodies, or in the fact that it followed the wish of Him who brought the disease into the world.

Procopius, History of the Wars

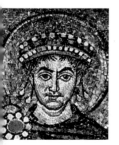

The Byzantine emperor Justinian

or cure the disease, many people promptly turned to religion for solace.

When plague returned as the Black Death in the middle of the 14th century, many Christians saw it as a latter-day Flood, the Almighty's way of stripping the world of sinners and punishing humankind for its wrongdoing. In 1348, the Italian writer Giovanni Boccaccio said of the Black Death

There came... a deadly pestilence... either because of the operations of the heavenly bodies, or because of the just wrath of God mandating punishment for our iniquitous ways.

During this and later outbreaks of plague, the devout resorted to self-immolation and the persecution of those whom they considered ungodly, for surely rooting out the source of sin would end the

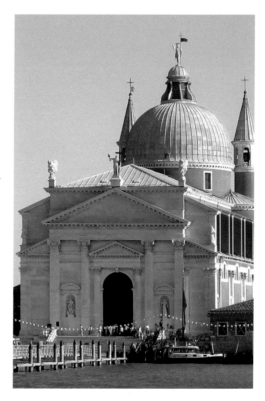

The striking Chiesa del Santissimo Redentore in Venice was built in the hope of halting a plague in 1576–7

punishment? Jews and Muslims were amongst those who were singled out as scapegoats and victimized for bringing the plague. In later centuries it was common to build or dedicate churches to God in the hope of appeasing Him and ending a plague. When Venice was struck by the plague in 1576, the Doge made a deal with God – the city would build the church of Redentore if God would end the plague. God did not rapidly honour the bargain: nine months passed and 50,000 people died before the plague was declared over. A festival celebrating the eventual end of the plague is still held every year on the third Sunday in July.

PLAGUES AND PLAYS

The Oberammergau Passion Play is performed every ten years in the German town of Oberammergau, in fulfilment of a promise made by the people of the town in 1633. They vowed to put on a religious play each decade if God spared them from the plague that was raging around the region. The deal seemed to work: the death rate fell from 20 in March 1633 to only one in July. It never reached the terrifying levels experienced elsewhere. The town now enjoys a healthy income from international visitors to the plays.

GOD'S VENGEANCE IN MAN'S HANDS

When humankind encounters something terrifyingly dangerous, a common response is to use it against others. Plague is no exception. The first documented use of plague as a weapon was in Kaffa in 1346 when the besieging Tartar army catapulted the corpses of plague victims over the city walls in order to infect the inhabitants. It was used more recently by the Japanese army in the Second World War: they hurled porcelain pots stuffed with plague-infected fleas into Chinese cities, causing thousands of cases of plague. The United States army is rumoured to have prepared plague as a weapon after the Second World War and the USSR produced an extremely virulent, antibiotic-resistant strain of the plague bacillus at bioweapons laboratories in Obolensk and Novosibirsk.

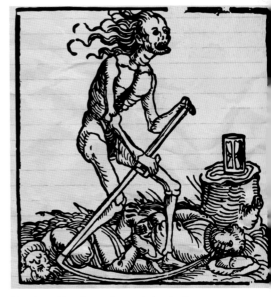

Death scything down plague victims in the 14th century

'Bad air'

While the popular and religious medieval view was that some diseases were inflicted directly and deliberately by God, the medical profession attempted to provide a more scientific explanation. Even so, this did not necessarily rule out the hand of God – it just explained how God's will manifested itself. There was, too, a belief that while God produced epidemics He was not particularly implicated in individual cases of illness. These were related to proximate causes over which victims had a varying degree of control.

An early and enduring explanation was that some form of balance or flow in the body had been disrupted. Models of the body which depend on balance are usually holistic and they produce a model of disease in which the causes of sickness are internal. According to these models, illness is caused by the body itself and it is cured by addressing the imbalance within it. Some aspects of modern medical science fit this model; the biochemical balance of the body can produce conditions with an entirely internal cause, which can be remedied by rebalancing the body's chemistry. The first suggested external source of disease, other than a divine agent, was 'miasma', or poisonous air.

The miasmatic model of disease can be traced back to the Hippocratic suggestion that heat leads to the putrefaction of vegetable and plant matter, which in turn produces noxious vapours or miasmas – leading to terrible fevers in humans. Malaria, which means 'bad air' in Italian, was believed for a long time to be the result of evil fumes from the swampy lands where

it was endemic. Many other tropical diseases were also thought to be caused by noxious air. From the Middle Ages onwards many of the measures taken against plague throughout Europe and the Middle East were designed to purify the air, replace bad air with good or avoid polluted air altogether. People left windows open to let in cool air and closed them against warm air; they burned scented woods and incense and carried posies of scented flowers or pungent plants such as onion or garlic. Plague doctors wore long, beaked masks containing strong-smelling herbs which they hoped would protect them from the miasma, as well as masking the stink of rotting flesh.

The miasmatic theory was predominant in Europe from the 18th century until the end of the 19th century. In 1854, *The Times* reported

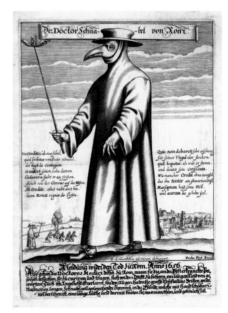

The plague doctors of Renaissance Europe looked suitably alarming in their protective garb

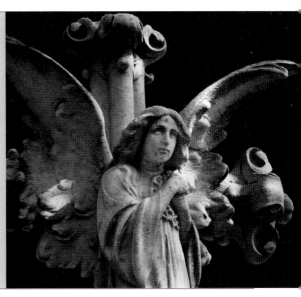

THE ANGEL OF DEATH

In the Tenth Annual Report of the Registrar General (1847), William Farr described the putrid air of London as

This disease-mist, arising from the breath of two millions of people, from open sewers and cholera... At another it carries fever on its wings. Like an angel of death it has hovered for centuries over London. But it may be driven away by legislation.

that the installation of new sewage works

... must have disturbed the soil, saturated with the remains of persons deposited here during the great plague [of 1665]... A deadly miasmatic atmosphere has been for some months arising... poisoning the surrounding atmosphere and causing an epidemic of cholera.

The determination to blame first plague and later cholera on miasmas hampered the development of the public health measures that might have alleviated epidemics. This way of thinking was most detrimental in the case of cholera because miasmists repeatedly rejected the recommendations of John Snow, who suggested that polluted water was the source of infection during the epidemics of the 1850s. As a result, tens of thousands of people died unnecessarily.

Of course, there is a sense in which 'bad air' really can cause illness and disease.

The famous smogs of 19th-century London and 20th-century China were heavy with pollutants and caused lung and chest conditions in the people who were forced to live in them. Factors such as pollution around factories, chemicals sprayed on to crops and even electromagnetic radiation from telecommunications have recently been blamed, rightly or wrongly, for clusters of illness ranging from asthma to leukaemia. The fallout from the nuclear accident at the Chernobyl nuclear power plant in the Ukraine in 1986, which had both immediate and long-term effects on the health of people living downwind of the reactor, would have looked very like miasmatic influence to earlier generations. Today, though, we distinguish between different types of 'bad air'. It could be polluted with toxic chemicals, or it might carry radiation or airborne microbes – the agents of disease that eluded discovery for centuries.

Agents of disease

People have been aware for millennia that some diseases are contagious (passed from one person to another) while others are not. Babylonian clay tablets from 1700BC show that people already knew that some skin diseases are contagious and some are not, though

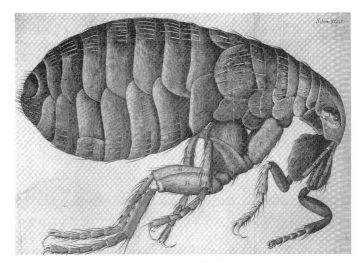

A flea can carry many diseases, including the plague

they had no explanation for the difference.

The idea that a disease might be caused by an external agent that is not supernatural first emerged some two thousand years ago, but there was no way of investigating it. Since then, we have discovered many kinds of microscopic agents of disease – and some larger ones, in the form of parasites and animal carriers – that finally explain how a disease might be 'catching'.

GERM THEORY AND CONTAGION

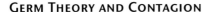

Most diseases, we now know, are caused by microscopic agents such as bacteria or viruses, but only the development of the optical and then the electron microscope has enabled us to investigate these tiny troublemakers. Long ago, some forward-looking scientists suspected that there was more to disease than meets the eye. Writing as far back as 36BC, the Roman author of *On Agriculture*, Marcus Terentius Varro, was on the right lines when he reported his suspicion that

... there are bred certain minute creatures which cannot be seen by the eyes, which float in the air and enter the body through the mouth and nose and there cause serious diseases.

Sadly, Varro had no way of verifying his belief.

Other scholars noted that there was a tendency for people to contract diseases if they attended sick patients or lived in close proximity with them – but that it did not always happen. Galen (AD129–c.216) and his followers decided that a person's humoral balance could predispose them to develop an illness that they were exposed to, an explanation that successfully fitted observation to their model of disease. In this way, a humoral model and a miasmatic model could just about jog along together, with the miasma bringing diseases that those prone to them would then develop.

Nearly a thousand years after Varro, Arab scholars pondered the idea that

ATHANASIUS KIRCHER (1602–80)

A German Jesuit polymath, Kircher was born in Geisa, Buchonia (near modern-day Hesse). He attended university in Paderborn but in 1622 the approaching Protestant forces forced him to flee to Köln. Although he fell through the ice crossing the frozen river Rhine he survived to have a glittering career as a professor, geologist, linguist, mathematician and student of medicine, physics, geology and Egyptology. He was one of the last Renaissance men – someone who could plausibly aspire to know everything that was known during his lifetime while being capable of adding to the body of knowledge.

He is considered to be the originator of Egyptology, even if the greater part of his work in the field eventually proved to be wrong. While in charge of erecting obelisks in Rome he sometimes added his own made-up hieroglyphs in the blank spaces, confounding later scholars. On a visit to southern Italy in 1638 he had himself lowered into the crater of Vesuvius, which was about to erupt at the time. On another occasion, he postulated that the tides are caused by water moving to and from a great underground ocean and that there are fires within the earth. He was also interested in fossils, recognizing some as the remains of animals that had turned to stone, and he invented the megaphone. His work in medicine was forward looking: he examined the blood of plague victims and declared the disease to be caused by tiny 'animalcules' (which might well have been blood cells). He advocated various methods of preventing the spread of disease, including isolating sufferers, quarantine, wearing facemasks and burning the clothes of victims.

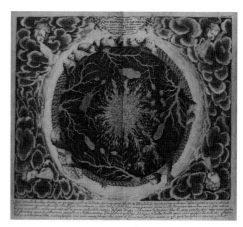

Kircher's model of the Earth gave it a fiery centre; the inner core is now thought to be around 7,000°C

diseases might be passed from one person to another, but there was a problem reconciling the model with Muslim beliefs. The Qu'ran taught that all illness came from God; but on the other hand, Mohammed had instructed followers to flee lepers 'as you would flee a lion', thereby suggesting that sickness could be avoided.

Ibn Qutayba's solution, in the 9th century, was to claim that epidemics were sent by God and were inescapable but that isolated cases of chronic conditions could be passed from person to person, so contagion could be avoided. In around 1020, Avicenna (Ibn Sina) tried to stop the transmission of disease by introducing a form of quarantine that would separate infected people from the healthy. He identified nine diseases that he considered contagious.

During the Black Death epidemic in the 14th century, the Arab physicians Ibn Khatima and Ibn al-Khatib suggested that some kind of 'contagious entity' entered the body and brought disease. A more precise formulation of something approaching germ theory was made in the 15th century by Girolamo Fracastoro, the Italian physician who first described and named syphilis. His 1546 treatise *De contagionibus et contagiosis morbis et earum curatione (On contagion and contagious diseases)* suggested that epidemic diseases were caused by living agents that were too small to see. They could be transmitted between people by (amongst other

methods) physical touch. He considered both plague and smallpox to be contagious in this way, but also believed that the influence of the stars was very important in directing the course of an epidemic.

TEEMING MULTITUDES

The invention of the microscope in the late 1500s revealed the teeming world of micro-organisms. Leeuwenhoek and Hooke brought micro-organisms to the attention of the scientific world, but they did not suggest that any of the tiny 'animalcules' caused disease. One of the first people to contemplate the link with disease was the German Jesuit scholar Athanasius Kircher, a polymath who used a microscope to examine the blood of plague victims in 1646. He found something that looked to

LOUIS PASTEUR (1822–95)

Born the son of a tanner in the Jura mountains, Pasteur trained as a chemist and became a professor at the University of Lille. His department was involved in solving practical problems for local industries. Pasteur's own interest was in the process of fermentation. He showed experimentally that the widely held belief in spontaneous generation was incorrect. He demonstrated that fermentation and spoiling in foods and liquids were the work of bacteria and that these bacteria could be killed by heating. Convinced that disease is caused by micro-organisms, he proved his theory by eradicating disease in silkworms, a problem that was devastating the French silk industry. When he created his first vaccine, against anthrax, he tested it in a spectacular experiment. Starting with two groups of sheep, he inoculated one group but not the other – then he injected both groups with live anthrax. When the sheep were inspected soon afterwards, all of the vaccinated animals were healthy but the others were dead or dying. The Institut Pasteur in Paris was founded in 1888 for the treatment of disease, and Pasteur was director until his death in 1895. As a national hero he was given a state funeral. His body lies in the Pantheon.

KOCH'S POSTULATES: LINKING MICROBES AND DISEASE

Koch's postulates are the rules for deciding whether a bacterium causes a disease. He stated that if an organism causes a disease it must:

- Be found in all cases of the disease
- Be capable of being grown as a pure culture
- Produce the original disease when introduced from the culture into a host
- Be retrievable from an inoculated animal and be capable of being cultured again.

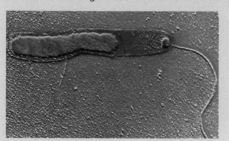

The water-borne bacterium vibrio cholerae, *which causes cholera in humans*

him like small worms and concluded that they caused the disease.

Even this was not enough to overthrow the dominant humoral and miasmatic models of disease. It was left to Louis Pasteur (1822–95) to forge a link between microbes and contagion. In a series of experiments he showed that fermentation, infection and putrefaction are caused by the presence of microbes – and that their progress can be halted by killing them with heat. Working with flasks of broth he showed that if a sealed flask was boiled the contents would not spoil, because the microbes it contained had been killed. If the broth was not boiled, or was left exposed to the air (allowing further contamination), the broth would spoil. Pasteur became a national hero by saving the French wine industry – his process of pasteurization (heat treatment) prevented wine from souring by killing the micro-organisms within it.

Pasteur made an important connection, but it was very general – anonymous microbes can cause disease. Robert Koch (1843–1910) went further by establishing

THE FIRST BACILLUS IDENTIFIED

Casimir Davaine (1812–82) first showed that anthrax passes directly from one cow to another. Robert Koch took up the study of the disease by isolating the bacillus from blood samples and then growing cultures. He demonstrated that although the bacillus can only survive for a short time outside a host, it produces endospores which can survive over a long period, remaining viable. It is the preservation of endospores in the soil that accounts for apparently spontaneous outbreaks of anthrax in uninfected herds of cattle, while the live bacillus transmits the disease between animals.

CONQUERING GERMS

Even before the definitive work of Pasteur and Koch, some medical scientists had stumbled across the link between microbial agents, infection and the methods for preventing infection. Working in Vienna General Hospital in 1848, Ignaz Semmelweis was shocked that the rates of death from puerperal fever (childbed fever) in newly-delivered mothers were much higher in a ward run by medical men than in a second ward run by midwives. Noticing that the doctors came straight from performing autopsies and post-mortems to delivering babies, he concluded that this was somehow the source of infection. After Semmelweis had introduced a rule that the doctors must wash their hands in a solution of chlorinated lime (calcium hypochlorite) before entering the delivery ward, the mortality rate fell to the level in the midwives' ward. Sadly, the implication that

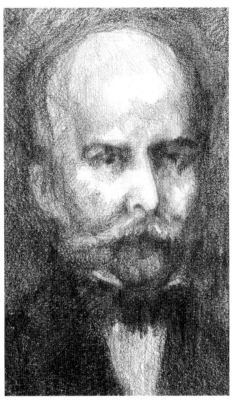

Ignaz Semmelweis' work should have changed the world – but, sadly, it received little attention outside Vienna

that each separate disease is caused by a specific microbe. In 1876 he identified the bacillus responsible for anthrax and then went on to discover the agents that cause tuberculosis and cholera. The cholera bacillus had in fact been isolated by the Italian Filippo Pacini in 1854, but his discovery was ignored because the miasmatic theory of disease was predominant at the time. However, his work was recognized in 1965 – the cholera bacterium was renamed as *Vibrio cholerae Pacini 1854.*

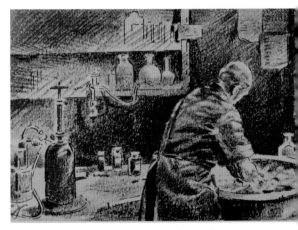

Preventing the spread of germs: Ignaz Semmelweis washing his hands before surgery. His theory was met with ridicule at the time

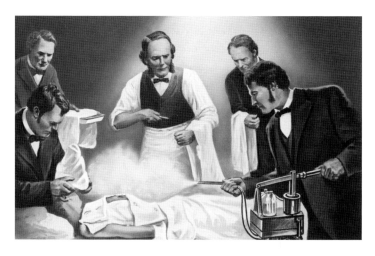

Lister's carbolic spray reduced the incidence of post-operative infection in his patients

doctors were spreading infection was so unpopular that Semmelweis' discovery was met with scorn and derision, so it made no significant impact outside his own hospital. Broken and frustrated, he left Vienna in 1850 and ended his days in a lunatic asylum.

The British surgeon Joseph Lister (1827–1912) was more successful. In 1869, he introduced a carbolic acid spray during operations and found that the incidence of post-operative . infection dropped considerably (see p.159). Lister knew that carbolic acid was used as an antiseptic for cleaning out the sewers in Carlisle and so he surmised that it would similarly kill disease in the operating theatre. He first tried carbolic acid by applying it in undiluted form to a young boy's serious leg injury. The boy's wound healed without infection, sparing him an amputation – an astonishing achievement at the time. Lister was widely mocked for his belief in 'invisible' germs, but the success he achieved won other doctors over to his methods.

The Black Death: reprise

There have been three great plague pandemics: the Plague of Justinian, which appeared in 541–2, the Black Death which lasted from 1346 to 1353, and a third pandemic that began in the Far East in 1792 and took a real hold in the 1850s. Continuing until 1959, it perhaps killed 25 million people. It was during this final pandemic that the means of transmission was finally understood and the disease could at last be tackled with confidence using antibiotics.

When the third pandemic of plague spread to Hong Kong in 1894, two rival research teams raced to identify the bacillus that was responsible. The Swiss-born Alexandre Yersin led one team and the Japanese scientist Shibasaburo Kitasato led the other. Both had previously been students of Robert Koch. Yersin worked in a straw hut with only a microscope and an autoclave, while Kitasato had a well-equipped hospital laboratory, yet it was Yersin who isolated the plague bacillus, now called *Yersinia pestis*. Yersin took seriously the connection the locals made between rats and plague and proved that the bacillus passes through the rodent host. He suspected a link with insects, but it was the French researcher Paul-Louis Simond who discovered the role of fleas in 1898. His research was dismissed, though: the British Indian Plague Research Commission considered his evidence 'to be hardly deserving of consideration' and declared that 'plague infected fleas are of no practical importance in regard to the spread of plague'. Over the next 30 years plague erupted and raged unchecked in India, killing 12.5 million people. In 1914, the British researchers A.W. Bacot and C.J. Martin finally confirmed Simond's theory by showing that the bacilli reproduce in the flea's foregut. The clump of bacteria causes a blockage, so when the flea tries to take its next meal of blood from a human host it effectively overflows: blood and bacilli are regurgitated into the victim, causing a new case of plague.

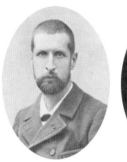 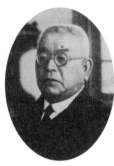

Alexandre Yersin (left) and Shibasaburo Kitasato (right) both strove to find the cause of plague

Viruses: tiny villains

While bacteria are microscopic, they are nowhere near as small as viruses. Viruses exist on the border between living and non-living things. They are little more than rogue proteins, but they are responsible for some of the deadliest diseases known. They can only survive and multiply inside a host cell, so they can't lie around for years like the time-bomb of anthrax endospores. Instead they need a reservoir – a population in which they can lurk, causing little harm, for years or even centuries. Often, the reservoir is an animal species.

The first clue to the existence of viruses came from Pasteur himself. Unable to find a bacterium responsible for rabies he suggested that there might be an even smaller germ that could not be seen with the microscope. (He did, nevertheless, manage to create a vaccine that was effective against the rabies virus.) Confirmation of the existence of these ultra-tiny agents of disease came in 1895. Working on the tobacco mosaic virus, the Dutch botanist Martinus Beijerinck discovered that he could take sap from an infected plant, pass it through the

The black rat is host to the fleas that carry the Yersinia pestis *bacillus – the cause of plague*

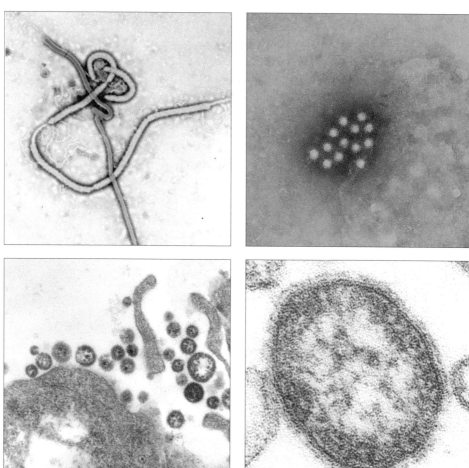

The agents of disease viewed under the microscope (clockwise from top left): Ebola fever, hepatitis A, measles and Lassa fever

finest porcelain filter and still infect other plants with it. A bacterium, he knew, would be stopped by the filter. He found that neither chemical action nor heat treatment made the infected sap ineffective, although the agent of contagion could not be grown on a culture medium. Even so, it was not an inert chemical toxin because it could apparently multiply. The infected sap could infect another plant and that could infect further plants. Beijerinck called his new agent of disease a 'virus', from the Latin name for poison. He published his findings in 1898. In the same year Friedrich Loeffler and Paul Frosch discovered the virus responsible for foot and mouth disease in cattle. The first human virus to be identified was the yellow fever virus in 1901. Beijerinck

had identified the cause of some of the deadliest diseases, including smallpox, rabies, polio and AIDS. However, viruses could not be examined until the electron microscope was invented in 1931.

What's eating you?

Some conditions are caused by agents much larger than bacteria and viruses. A parasite is an organism that lives in or on another living entity. Parasites in humans range from tapeworms that live in the gut and can be several metres long, to tiny protozoa that hide in the blood cells. A tapeworm is visible to the naked eye when it is expelled, as are many of the other worms and mites that live in the human body. Even so, people in the past have not always made the connection between particular symptoms and the presence of a parasite. Some medical thinkers have even postulated parasites where there are none, such as the 'tooth worms' thought to have caused tooth decay. Many ancient Egyptian hieroglyphs for diseases end with the worm determinant, suggesting that they considered a worm responsible for the ailment.

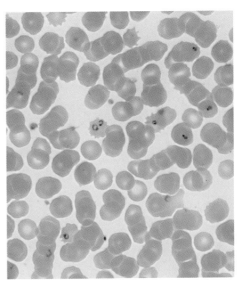

Plasmodium is responsible for causing malaria, which kills a million people every year

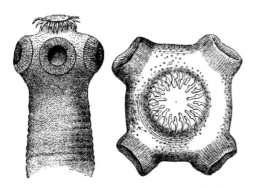

The pork tapeworm has four suckers on its 'head', clearly visible in views from the side and above

Circumstantial evidence often led thoughtful physicians and philosophers to ponder how disease was spread. Indian physicians established a link between rats and bubonic plague long before the flea was identified as a carrier. In Europe, malaria was blamed on miasmas from marshy land, but in India a link with mosquitoes had been made as early as the 6th century BC – the time of Susruta, the great physician. The first scientific discovery of a link between parasites and disease was made by Ibn Zuhr (Avenzoar, 1091–1161) in 12th-century Moorish Spain. Ibn Zuhr introduced experimental method into surgery and developed methods of dissection and autopsy that led him to the discovery that scabies is caused by a parasite.

Some parasites are microscopic and others remain hidden in the body. They can cause illness by producing toxins or by

BUILDING THE PANAMA CANAL

Yellow fever decimated the troops during the American–Spanish war in Cuba (1898–1901). In the 1800s, yellow fever and malaria caused so many deaths on the French project to build the Panama canal that was to join the Atlantic and Pacific Oceans that the venture was abandoned. A Cuban physician, Carlos Finlay, established a link between yellow fever and mosquitoes with a rather unethical experiment that involved allowing mosquitoes to first bite yellow fever victims and then healthy individuals (who did not stay healthy for long). A massive programme of mosquito eradication began, which was organized by the US Army Yellow Fever Commission. The Commission drained the swamps where the mosquitoes bred, fitted buildings with screens, cut back grass and poured oil or chemicals on to the edges of ponds to kill mosquito larvae. Yellow fever was eradicated completely and the incidence of malaria decreased considerably, allowing the canal to be completed in 1914.

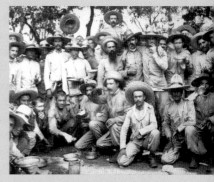

Prisoners and soldiers of the American-Spanish war fell victim to many kinds of fever

diverting the nourishment the body needs. Malaria is caused by the plasmodium parasite, which is passed between people by the *Anopheles* mosquito. Humans are injected with infected blood which travels to the liver and enters the bloodstream. The plasmodium parasite multiplies inside the blood cells which then burst, releasing more plasmodium. Although Susruta knew that the mosquito spreads malaria, he was not aware that the real culprit is the plasmodium parasite.

The idea that disease could be caused by parasites and carried by insects did not emerge until 1866, when Patrick Manson, a Scots physician, was working on an island off the southeast coast of China. His study of elephantiasis, which causes a disfiguring swelling of the limbs and genitals, revealed that the disease is caused by a parasitic worm that is introduced by the bite of a mosquito. It soon emerged

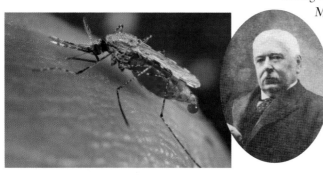

Mosquitos can transmit many diseases, including malaria, yellow fever and elephantiasis – a disease researched by Patrick Manson (right)

that other tropical diseases are caused by parasites, including dysentery (an amoeba), sleeping sickness (a protozoan) and schistosomiasis (a worm). The puzzle of malaria, the greatest killer of all, was solved by Ronald Ross while he was working in the Indian Medical Service. After realizing, in 1894, that mosquito bites were implicated in the development of malaria, he discovered the malaria parasite in the gut of the *Anopheles* mosquito and related the lifecycle of the protozoan to the disease. In 1901 he received the Nobel Prize for his work.

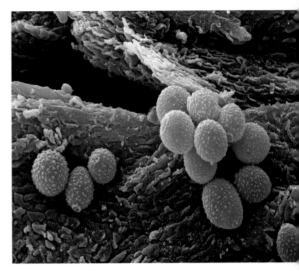

Spores of the fungus which causes athlete's foot

Magic mushrooms?

To most people fungi are mushrooms and toadstools but there are many microscopic fungi, some of which cause disease in humans. Fungal infections are not the most glamorous of diseases, but they are widespread – athlete's foot, or *tinea pedis*, is one of the most common diseases in the world. The first description of a human disease caused by a fungus is in the Indian Vedic texts (c.2000–c.1000BC) in which mycetoma presents as 'padavalmika' ('foot anthill'), but a link with a fungus was not made for thousands of years.

Fungi were, in fact, the first microbes to be found guilty of causing disease. In 1835, Italian lawyer and farmer Agostino Bassi discovered that an epidemic disease of silkworms was caused by a fungus. Then between 1837 and 1841, the Hungarian David Gruby and the Polish/German Robert Remak discovered *tinea favosa*, the first known mycotic disease in humans. Gruby went on to identify *Candida albicans*, the fungus that causes thrush, in

1842. But attention soon passed to the more interesting bacteria and viruses, and fungi were largely neglected until the 1890s. Interest in fungal infections has enjoyed something of a renaissance since the rise in immunosuppressive conditions, which allow opportunistic infection by fungi. HIV/AIDS sufferers and transplant patients taking immuno-suppressive drugs are particularly susceptible to fungal infections.

Disease on the brain

Prions are the most recently discovered microscopic agents of disease. A small group of diseases affecting the brain and the nervous system puzzled scientists for years: they proved resistant to all forms of antibiotic and were not affected by ultraviolet light, which would destroy a virus. These diseases include scrapie, a disease of sheep, BSE (Bovine Spongiform Encephalopathy or 'mad cow disease') and

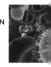

CJD (Creutzfeldt-Jakob Disease). All result in degeneration of the brain to a spongy mass, accompanied by gradual loss of brain function. In 1982, American biologist Stanley Prusiner suggested that the culprit is a proteinaceous infectious particle, or 'prion'. A prion is not a microbe but is an abnormal form of a protein found naturally in the body. When it comes into contact with the normal form, it can corrupt it. The abnormality spreads, slowly destroying brain tissue.

In the 1980s, an epidemic of BSE was caused by feeding cattle with infected protein in meal derived from animal carcasses. It led to 164 human deaths (to May 2009) from variant CJD, the result of eating nerve fibres from infected cattle (typically, minced up in hamburgers and other processed foods). As CJD has an

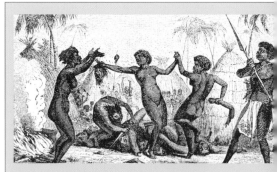

Tales of cannibalism have been connected with many societies, but in the case of the Fore eating dead relatives caused more than a PR problem

DON'T EAT DEAD PEOPLE

A horrible disease reached epidemic proportions amongst the Fore people of Papua New Guinea in the late 1950s. Called kuru, it produced headaches, joint pain, shaking and eventual death and it was particularly common amongst women and children. The American physician Daniel Carleton Gajdusek (b.1923) studied the disease and discovered a link with funerary cannibalism. The Fore people had a custom of eating their dead relatives (including the brains) as a way of restoring the vital spirit of the deceased to the community. Generally, the men preferred to eat pork and this seems to have been a wise choice. Although just eating a well-cooked ancestor should not result in kuru, preparing the meal is a likely source of infection and this task fell to the women. When the ruling Australian authorities outlawed cannibalism and Christian missionaries campaigned against it, the incidence of kuru fell. Gajdusek worked before the discovery of prions, so he could not explain how the disease was transmitted.

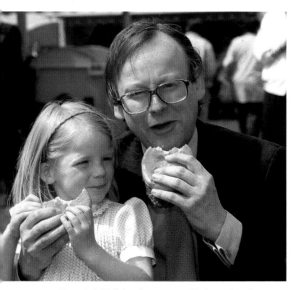

British MP John Gummer publicly ate hamburgers with his young daughter to demonstrate his belief that British beef carried no health risk

incubation period of years, or even decades, new cases are still coming to light.

Passing it on

It has long been clear, from common sense and everyday observation, that children inherit characteristics from their parents, but the mechanism was not revealed until 1865. The work of Austrian monk Gregor Mendel (1822–84) established that the characteristics of a child are inherited from its parents in the form of mixed pairs of genes, one from each parent. Some of the genetic information might make a person susceptible to disease or it might cause a particular inherited condition. Cystic fibrosis (CF) and Huntington's chorea are both caused by faulty genes. A child needs to gain a CF gene from each parent in order to develop cystic fibrosis, but Huntington's chorea requires only one faulty gene. If a parent suffers from Huntington's chorea, the child has a 50 per cent chance of inheriting the condition.

PARENTS AND PEAS

Basing his research on pea plants, Gregor Mendel used probability theory and quantitative methods to solve the mystery of inheritance. He found that if he crossed a plant bearing white flowers with one bearing purple flowers, all of the offspring produced purple flowers. If he then bred from the offspring, one in four produced white flowers. From this he deduced that there is a 'factor' (as he called it) inherited

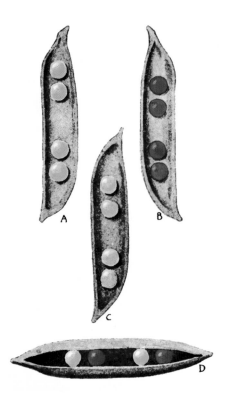

Between 1856 and 1863, Mendel carried out his experiments in genetics using peas. The significance of his work was only recognized in the 20th century

from each parent. Purple flowers were dominant, so if a plant had one factor for purple flowers (or gene, as we would call it now) it would produce purple flowers. It would only produce white flowers if it had two factors for white. Mendel was able to work out the mechanism of inheritance because he turned to mathematics after noticing the 3:1 ratio. He also worked with a single discrete feature – purple or white flowers – rather than a variable feature such as height.

The English physician Sir Archibald Garrod (1857–1936) combined the new

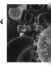

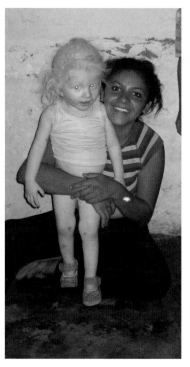

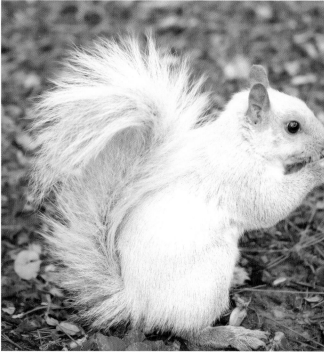

Albinos – whether people or animals – have no coloured pigments in their bodies. Only 1 in 17,000 humans is affected by albinism, although 1 in 70 is a carrier of the gene

knowledge of Mendelian inheritance with chemical techniques when he examined metabolism and disease in an extended study of several families who were suffering from a genetic disorder. He realized that the previously unknown causes of many diseases might be explained in terms of inherited metabolic disorders. He pioneered the idea of one gene coding for one enzyme and showed that most hereditary enzyme defects are recessive. The most well-known condition he investigated was albinism, in which the body's inability to make pigments leads to white-blond(e) hair and very pale skin. Garrod first presented his work in 1908 but he continued to expand upon it throughout his life.

Although Mendel worked out his model of inheritance in 1865 it took until 1911 for the mechanism, involving chromosomes and genes, to be properly understood. The first work identifying specific genes for particular characteristics (in fruit flies) was carried out by a team at Columbia University, New York.

It laid the foundations for gene mapping and, ultimately, the project to map the whole of the human genome, which began in 1990. The mapping of the genome is revealing more and more about which genes are responsible for certain disorders. It offers the hope that at some point in the future we might be able to 'fix' some of the

HAEMOPHILIA: THE ROYAL DISEASE

Haemophilia is a genetic condition in which the blood fails to clot because a clotting agent is missing. In haemophilia A, the most common form of the disease, the missing clotting agent is Factor VIII and in haemophilia B it is Factor IX. When haemophiliacs are cut or bruised, their blood continues to flow without stopping so they readily bleed to death. Before modern times sufferers have rarely reached adulthood. Haemophilia is usually carried by the female line and inherited by male children, but it can also occur as a random genetic mutation in a family with no history of haemophilia. In rare cases it can be acquired in later life. Gene therapy might one day provide a treatment for the condition.

Haemophilia famously affected a number of European royals during the 19th and 20th centuries, beginning with Queen Victoria's eighth child, Prince Leopold. The royal family blamed a curse that had been supposedly cast on the Coburg family by an angry monk. He was thought to have been taking revenge for the marriage of the young princess Antoinette de Kohary to a Coburg prince. The practice of intermarriage among the European royal families led to the disease popping up all over Europe. One victim was Tsarevich Alexei, son

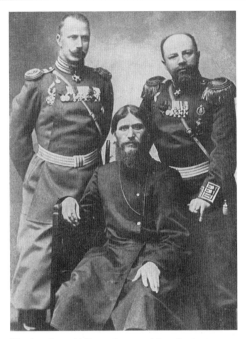

The 'mad monk' Rasputin, seated here between Colonel Loma and Prince Putianin, helped to bring down the Russian royal family

of Tsar Nikolai II. The tsarina believed that the 'mad monk' Rasputin could keep the boy's condition under control and as a result Rasputin came to exert considerable power over the royal family. This helped to pave the way for the Russian Revolution in 1917.

genes that either produce serious conditions or create a susceptibility to them.

While an understanding of the genetic transmission of some conditions might help us to eradicate or cure them, genetic engineering raises complex ethical issues. Is it legitimate to 'select out' people with autism, Down's syndrome or other genetic variations in order to come closer to a generally accepted ideal human form? At the extreme end of the spectrum, eugenicists hope that an understanding of genetics will enable us to perfect the human race. But this way of thinking

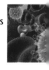

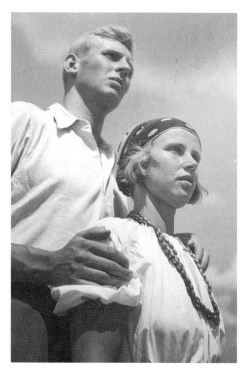

The Aryan ideal – tall, athletic, blond-haired and blue-eyed. The Nazis strove to maintain the purity of this 'race' through their eugenics programmes

Antoine Lavoisier (1743–94) and Justus von Liebig (1803–73) revealed the importance of chemical reactions in body processes. Respiration – that of the whole organism and at a cellular level – nutrition, and all other aspects of metabolism depend on the carefully balanced input and output of different chemicals, including vital nutrients. Liebig's studies of diet, and the ways in which the body works at a chemical level, led to the realization of the need for a balanced diet, providing the body with the

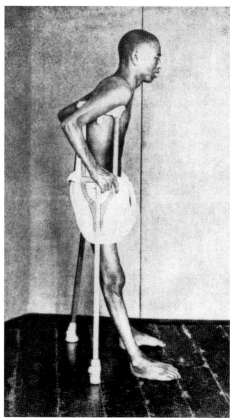

The effects of beriberi, caused by deficiency of vitamin B1 in the diet. Symptoms include weight loss, severe lethargy and even, in advanced cases, heart failure

underpinned the Nazis' perception of Aryan Germans as the 'master race' and allowed the Holocaust. Despite having had such a bad press, eugenics still has its proponents – most notably the biologist Francis Crick, one of the team who discovered the structure of DNA.

Chemical imbalances

The idea that the healthy body has a natural state of balance, while imbalance produces sickness, was not dispelled with the humours. The emerging biochemical model of the body led to a different concept of balance: one of chemical balance.

required quantities of different types of chemicals to maintain good health.

Some aspects of chemical balance are beyond our control, though. The body produces and uses enzymes (which act as catalysts in chemical reactions) and hormones (which act as chemical messengers). If these are not produced in the correct quantities, or are not recognized, serious illness can result.

Vital chemicals: vitamins

The human body needs tiny quantities of some chemicals (vitamins), although it is still not clear how some of these vitamins are used by the body. A lack of vitamins causes serious medical complications, some of which can be fatal.

The earliest vitamin deficiency-related illness to be studied and cured was scurvy, which results from a lack of vitamin C. First

SCURVY ON A VOYAGE ROUND THE WORLD

This disease is likewise usually attended with a strange dejection of the spirits, and with shiverings, tremblings, and a disposition to be seized with the most dreadful terrors on the slightest accident... But it is not easy to compleat the long roll of the various concomitants of this disease; for it often produced putrid fevers, pleurisies, the jaundice, and violent rheumatick pains and sometimes it occasioned an obstinate costiveness, which was generally attended with a difficulty of breathing; and this was esteemed the most deadly of all the scorbutick symptoms: at other times the whole body, but more especially the legs, were subject to ulcers of the worst kind, attended with rotten bones, and such a luxuriancy of fungous flesh, as yielded to no remedy... the tears of wounds, which had been for many years healed, were forced open again by this virulent distemper.

George Anson, *A Voyage Round the World in the Years 1740–44* (London, 1776)

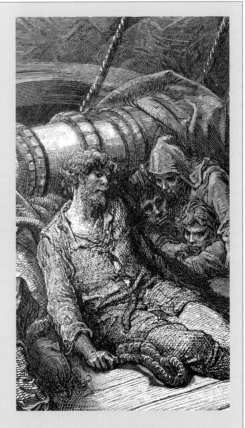

Scurvy – caused by a lack of vitamin C in the diet – plagued sailors who embarked on long voyages. Vitamin C is found in fresh fruit and vegetables

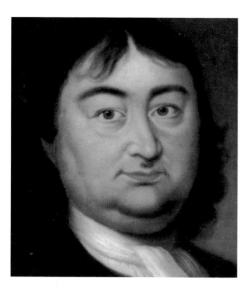

The logical conclusion? Vitus Bering, observing that the symptoms of scurvy disappeared once on land, was convinced that the cure lay in the earth itself

described by Hippocrates, it affected besieged cities and their besiegers for millennia and it was endemic among Crusaders in the 13th century. It became a particularly pressing problem from the 15th century onwards, though, when long sea journeys became increasingly common. The disease that Sir Richard Hawkins called

'the plague of the Sea, and the Spoyle of Mariners' produced terrible and often fatal effects. Symptoms included blackened skin, ulcers, respiratory distress, loss of teeth and the strange growth of extraneous gum tissue, which then rotted and stank. There were psychological effects, too. Sailors became extremely sensitive – they would cry out in agony at the scent of flowers or fruit, and the sound of gunshot was enough to kill a sufferer in the last stages of scurvy. Vasco da Gama lost two thirds of his crew on a journey to India in 1499, and 80 per cent of Magellan's crew died while he was crossing the Pacific in 1520.

Landfall was the salvation of sailors with scurvy, for there they could eat a normal diet again. Some, like the Dutch navigator Vitus Bering, thought that the mere presence of earth provided a cure for scurvy. He died half-buried in the ground, trying to cure his illness. Experienced sailors and ships' surgeons were aware that scurvy was cured by fresh fruit and vegetables and the so-called 'scurvy grass', but no-one knew

Many people use vitamin supplements in the hope of avoiding deficiencies

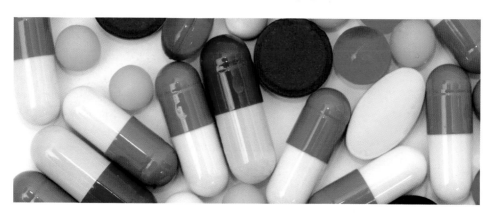

why. In 1617, the English surgeon John Woodall wrote of sailors who had been cured of scurvy by eating fresh citrus fruit and in 1734 the Dutch writer Johann Bachstrom wrote that 'scurvy is solely owing to a total abstinence from fresh vegetable food, and greens; which is alone the primary cause of the disease'. Yet scurvy continued to plague sailors until 1795, when the Admiralty issued citrus juice to all sailors in the Royal Navy, thereby eradicating the problem at a stroke.

Although citrus fruit had been found to cure scurvy, the cause of the disease was still unknown. The concept of vitamins emerged in 1912 when the Polish biochemist Casimir Funk proposed that tiny quantities of essential chemicals are needed in the diet, naming them vitamins for 'vital amines' (although they are not actually amines). With improved methods of chemical analysis, deficiency diseases could be explored in more detail. Vitamin C – ascorbic acid – was finally isolated between 1928 and 1933, independently by the efforts of Hungarian and American research teams.

Hormones: diabetes *mellitus*

Hormones act as messengers within the body. They help to keep track of aspects of the metabolism and they initiate, control and halt processes. The first hormonal disorder to be investigated was diabetes, in which the hormone insulin is either missing or is not recognized. The body is consequently not able to absorb sugar as it should but instead excretes it in the urine, so the level of sugar in the blood is not controlled.

An ancient Egyptian account of a rare disease that caused the sufferer to urinate frequently and lose weight rapidly is probably the first reference to diabetes. Diabetes (which means 'syphon' in Greek) was given its name by the Greek physician Aretaeus (fl.AD100), because of the way in which fluid passes through the diabetic body.

For fluids do not remain in the body, but use the body only as a channel through which they may flow out.

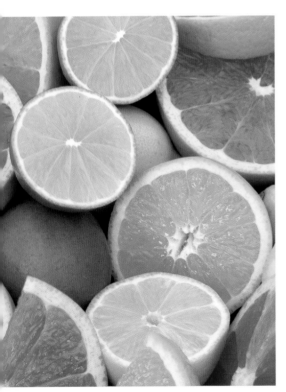

Citrus fruits were known to cure scurvy long before the chemical mechanism of the illness and its cure were understood

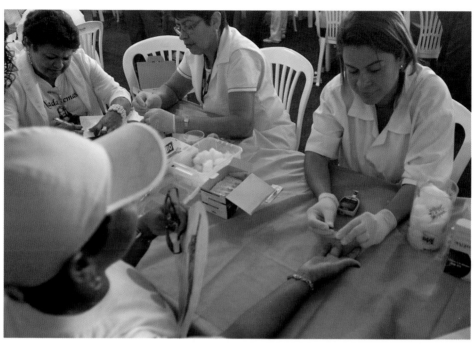

Sugarcoating the procedure: chemical testing for diabetes became commonplace in the 19th century, putting an end to the longstanding practice of tasting a patient's urine for signs of excess sugar in the bloodstream

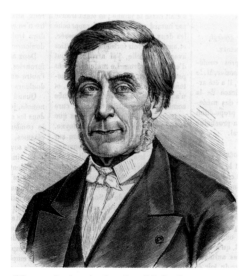

Often credited as the founder of diabetology, Apollinaire Bouchardat made advances in the understanding of diabetes and its treatment

Soon afterwards, Galen suggested that diabetes was a kidney disorder. Avicenna (c.980–1037) was the first physician to give a full description of the disease, which remained rare in his lifetime. The sweet taste of the urine, noticed by the English physician Thomas Willis in 1674, became the standard means of diagnosing diabetes *mellitus* – so called because mellitus means 'honey'. During the 19th century, chemical tests replaced the unsavoury practice of tasting the diabetic patient's urine, but the underlying cause of the disease was still not understood. The breakthrough came during the Franco-Prussian War (1870–1), when the French physician Apollinaire Bouchardat noticed that a reduced diet improved the condition of his diabetic patients. He went on to make a connection with calorie intake and also suggested that the pancreas might be at the root of the problem. In 1920, the American Moses Barron discovered the relationship of the pancreas to diabetes while conducting an autopsy on a diabetic subject. Frederick Banting then showed that the hormone insulin is produced by the islets of Langerhans in the pancreas, for which he shared the Nobel Prize for Physiology or Medicine in 1923.

Enzymes: getting things going

An enzyme is a protein that acts as a catalyst – it speeds up or facilitates a chemical reaction, but is not used up during the reaction. Enzymes are used in all cells and they play a part in all aspects of body chemistry. Without

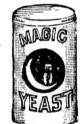

The action of enzymes produced by yeast causes fermentation

PORPHYRIA: MAD KINGS AND VAMPIRES?

The porphyrias are a group of conditions resulting from a deficiency of one or more of eight enzymes responsible for producing haem, the red pigment in blood. Symptoms of porphyria can include periods of madness, pale skin and aversion to sunlight. Some medical historians believe that the English king George III – 'Mad King George' – may have suffered from porphyria. It has also been connected with vampirism. Vampires, like porphyrics, are popularly thought to be pale and shun sunlight. Garlic, a food high in sulphur, is harmful to porphyrics and, of course, to vampires too. Porphyria was first properly described and named by the German Dr Schultz, in 1874. In 1930 Hans Fischer described haem as the compound that makes blood red and grass green.

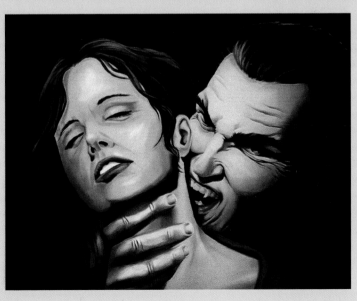

Vampires – but not porphyrics – like to bite people

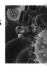

them, many chemical reactions upon which the body depends would happen too slowly or not at all, so an inability to produce or use enzymes can have a serious impact. For example, a person lacking some digestive enzymes might be unable to digest certain types of food.

When Pasteur discovered the role of yeast in fermentation he was not aware of the chemistry of the process, but he decided that it was catalysed by a vital force in the yeast. The role of an enzyme was discovered in 1897, when Eduard Buchner found that living yeast cells are not necessary to produce fermentation. In 1926, James B. Sumner first extracted and crystallized an enzyme, urease, in pure form.

Diseases of excess

Hippocrates knew that a balanced diet helped to keep the body healthy, and Milton's God has the archangel Michael tell Adam that humankind can avoid much disease by observing

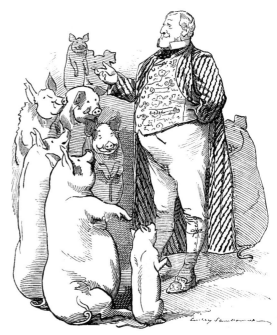

From the 18th century, there were enough obese people for them to become a source of humour

> The rule of 'Not too much' – by
> temperance taught,
> In what thou eatest and drinkest; seeking
> from thence
> Due nourishment, not gluttonous delight.

Despite this sound advice from the highest authorities, many people have overindulged whenever they have been able to do so. For thousands of years an excess of food and drink was seen as a sign of wealth, rather than just foolishness or greed. The ancient Romans, for example, held vast feasts at which they ate and drank so much that they

were often sick. But day-to-day indulgence has been limited to a privileged minority for much of history. It was not until the 18th century that diseases of excess started to have an impact on a significant number of people. Cartoonists lambasted fat, port-soaked gentlemen tormented by gout, and for the first time a substantial number of portraits depicted over-sized or obese individuals. Samuel Johnson records taking a 'simple' breakfast in the London town house of Margaret Dodds in 1776, where he was served oatmeal with sweet cream, smoked herrings, sardines with mustard sauce, grilled trout with white butter sauce, cold veal pies, grilled kidneys, sausages with mashed potatoes, beef tongue with hot horseradish sauce and 'enough bacon to feed a hungry army'. He was offered seven types of bread, with a choice of butter, honey, orange marmalade, raspberry jam, cherry jam and apple jam, all washed down with French and Spanish brandies, fresh apple cider, tea and coffee. It is hardly surprising that obesity was on the rise.

The body turns against itself

Rudolf Virchow (1821–1902) realized that cancers are produced by abnormal cells reproducing rapidly. The causes of many cancers are still not fully understood but some have a genetic element, many can be triggered by environmental and lifestyle factors, and others are caused by a virus. Normal cells divide in a controlled way. If some stimulus causes cell reproduction to go wrong, the resulting abnormal cells may make more and more copies of themselves. They are not attacked by the body's immune system as an invading organism would be.

Another way in which the body can go into overdrive and cause its own destruction is during the so-called cytokine storm response. This happens when the immune system attempts to destroy a virus or a bacterium by flooding the body with cytokines. Some infections can prompt the production of cytokines at such high levels that the body tissues are destroyed. This is one reason why the variant of flu that caused the 1918 pandemic was so deadly, and it also

The 'father of pathology', Dr Rudolf Virchow

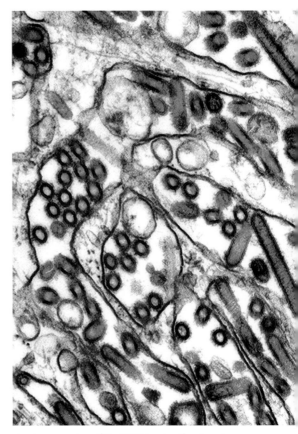

A microscope view of the H5N1 avian flu virus, here seen in green. The infection usually affects poultry, but can be transmitted to humans by direct contact

caused the high mortality rate among humans of the avian flu strain H5N1, which appeared in the Far East in 2003.

DEADLY FLU

The flu virus first came to humans thousands of years ago. It was transmitted from animals, probably pigs or birds, which are still sources of new strains of human flu. The earliest known mention of human flu is in the Hippocratic texts; the first known pandemic was in 1580, beginning in Asia and

PANDEMIC FLU IN BRAZIL, 1918

Rear Admiral William B. Caperton, of the United States Navy, described conditions in Rio de Janeiro, Brazil when his crew went ashore to bury their shipmates, who had died of flu in October 1918:

> *Conditions in the cemetery beggared description. Eight hundred bodies in all states of decomposition, and lying about in the cemetery, were awaiting burial. Thousands of buzzards swarmed overhead. In the city itself there were no longer medicines, or wood for coffins and very little food. Rich and poor alike were stricken. In the big public hospital which had the contract for burying the city's dead, hundreds of naked bodies lay thrown upon each other like cord wood and at least one instance was known of a live man being dragged out from the piles... Ashore, more than one thousand people died daily. Many of those whom we had known well and been fond of were carried off and the streets of Rio de Janeiro, generally gay and vivid with movement and color, were deserted and motionless.*

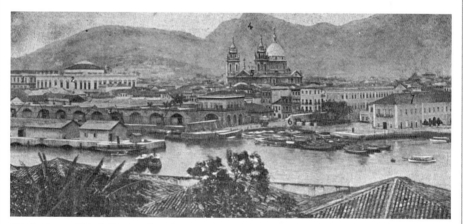

The harbour of Rio de Janeiro, Brazil, where Caperton's crew were greeted by an army of corpses during the flu pandemic of 1918

spreading to Europe. Flu epidemics have occurred frequently, and at irregular intervals, as the virus has mutated and people's immunity to it has no longer been effective. A particularly vicious strain of flu emerged at the end of the First World War: it was probably carried around the world by soldiers returning from the European front. It spread rapidly, first among military personnel living in crowded conditions and then among civilians who had contact with returning soldiers. The highest mortality rate was among the young and healthy, which confounded the medics – they were

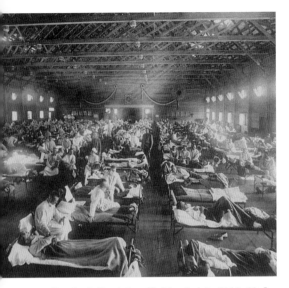

Pandemic flu victims filled hospitals in 1918–19. It was an unusually severe and deadly strain

for its tragic mortality rate. Research has involved exhuming samples of the virus from bodies buried in the permafrost of Alaska and then cloning it (not an entirely prudent course of action with a virus that was responsible for killing around 50 million people less than a hundred years ago). The DNA of the virus has been sequenced and the way in which it makes its way into human cells before it replicates and bursts out has been understood. But there is still no secure method of combating the virus or the cytokine storm it can generate.

All change

As human understanding and science have evolved, so has the predominant model of disease. People's belief in divine visitation, an imbalance of the body's humours or evil emanations from swamps and foul places has given way to a scientific model. We now know that diseases have many different causes: bacteria, viruses and protozoa; biochemical imbalances and malfunctions; genetic accident; the effects of an unhealthy lifestyle; bodily or substance abuse; and environmental factors such as pollution or toxins. We also know the causes of many diseases and their detailed biochemical effect on the body. But the key to some major diseases, such as cancer and many types of mental illness, has remained out of our reach.

accustomed to seeing children, the elderly and the sick fall victim to flu. Typically, a healthy patient's immune system launched a robust attack on the invading virus but then took its response to extremes, precipitating a cytokine storm that attacked the body itself, causing multiple organ failure. Victims often turned blue or black because there was no oxygenated blood reaching their skin. They drowned in their own blood as their lungs disintegrated. (If the immune system had not been strong enough to have produced a cytokine storm, the virus could have run riot and the patient might then have died of pneumonia.)

The 1918 H1N1 flu virus

Scientists are studying the 1918 flu virus in the hope of uncovering the reason

It is not only models of disease that change over time. Diseases themselves change – some old ones disappear or

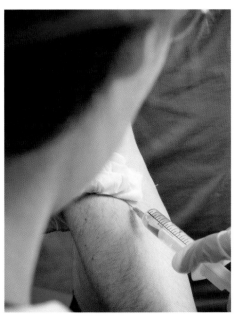

Thanks to medical advances, we can now treat many diseases that were previously deadly with a simple injection or course of pills

become less virulent while new ones emerge. For instance, contemporary accounts of a terrible plague that raged in and around Athens in the 5th century BC do not appear to match any diseases that we know today. Perhaps the Athenians were laid low by a disease that is no longer found. Diseases change – some quickly, and some more slowly – and they become more or less dangerous. Viral diseases change more quickly than bacterial diseases, because the replication of viruses is very rapid and prone to error. The high mutation rate in viruses makes it easy for them to adapt to new conditions and to infect new hosts – moving from pigs to humans, for example. The flu

vaccine must be re-engineered each year in order to keep up with the new features of the virus. Bacteria change, too, and can become resistant to the antibiotics with which we combat them. The idea that some diseases change and evolve, that they are organic entities in themselves, is a new addition to our model of disease. The Black Death, responsible for perhaps 50 million deaths in the Middle Ages, is traditionally considered to have been a mixture of bubonic, septicaemic and pneumonic plague. But some features of the symptoms, as well as the transmission pattern (as recorded in historical documents), are quite different from later incidences of plague. Some medical historians have questioned that it was plague at all. They have suggested that it might have been anthrax, a haemorrhagic fever similar to Ebola fever, or perhaps even a combination of diseases.

Various diseases have waxed and waned for reasons we cannot discover. Leprosy died out in Europe at around the time that plague arrived on the scene; cancer, asthma and many allergy-related conditions increased during the 20th century; plague did not return to Europe with any great virulence after the second pandemic. We are now confronting diseases that were undreamed of a century ago, including AIDS, Ebola fever, SARS and chronic fatigue syndrome. And we are still coming across new disease-causing agents, too – prions were only discovered in 1982. Who knows what other sources of illness will be discovered and to what extent we will have to adjust our model of disease in the future?

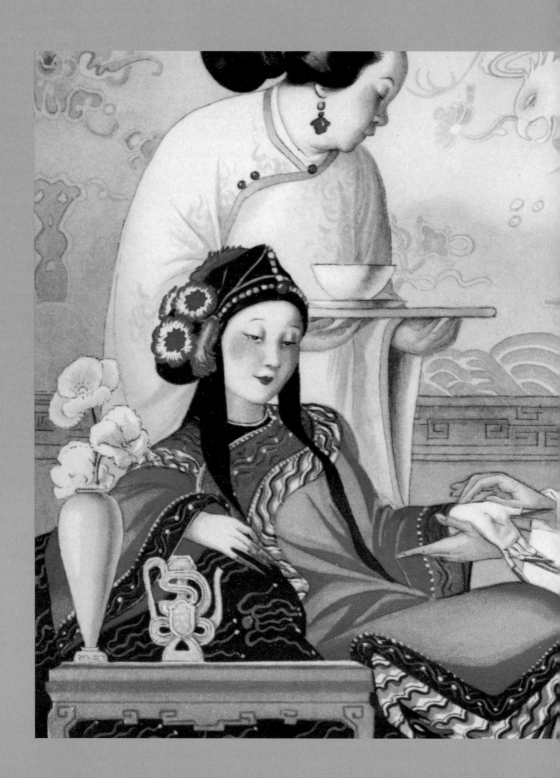

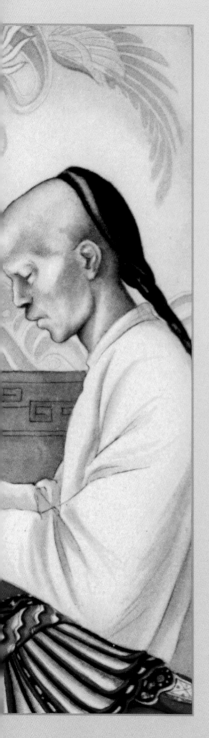

CHAPTER 3

DIAGNOSIS

For thousands of years, doctors examined patients with little hope of reaching a diagnosis or providing effective treatment. The best they could usually hope for was to predict whether a patient would live or die. Even if they could identify a condition there was rarely a cure, and some treatments made patients worse.

But over time, diagnostic techniques and tools have improved greatly. At first, doctors peered and poked, sniffed and tasted: then they developed instruments to help them listen and measure and record. Now doctors can look inside our bodies with relative ease. They can examine our bones, our brains and our organs without cutting us open, and use microscopes to investigate the smallest components of our bodies and search for the agents which cause disease. Improving diagnostic tools and techniques have developed alongside the evolving models of the human body and the diseases that afflict it. Without an understanding of the body and disease, no amount of measurements and observations will help the doctor to treat the patient. Yet along with knowledge and skill, the doctor brings compassion, concern and the shared humanity to draw from the patient embarrassing or frightening details which may be crucial to a diagnosis.

Taking the pulse has always been central to diagnosis in Chinese medicine

What's the problem?

If a patient goes to the doctor with a missing limb, a gaping wound or an ugly abscess, the nature of the problem is easy to see. But internal injuries and illnesses must have mystified early practitioners with little medical or anatomical knowledge. A patient might be vomiting or feverish or in pain for any number of reasons, but until very recently there has been no way of establishing the cause with confidence.

By recording symptoms (described by the patient) and signs (clinical indications measured or observed by the physician) doctors built up profiles of conditions even if they could not explain or treat them. From these records, they developed skills in diagnosis and prognosis (telling the patient what to expect). Many early doctors created astonishingly detailed descriptions of illnesses. Their observations were so accurate that we can often identify the conditions even now. The Edwin Smith papyrus from ancient Egypt gives a good account of quadriplegia, referring to the incontinence and the persistent erection caused by injury to the upper spine. Ancient Indian texts give accurate descriptions of diabetes, tuberculosis and smallpox, and Procopius' description of bubonic plague is entirely recognizable. But with no understanding of the underlying processes of an illness, early doctors could do little

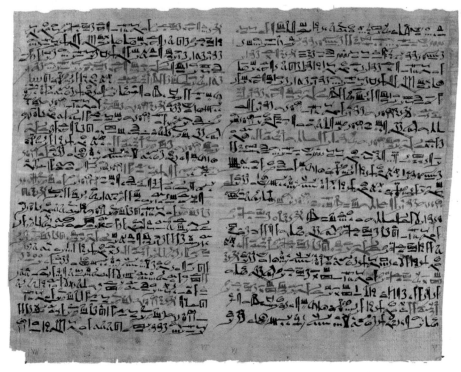

The Edwin Smith papyrus provides us with detailed records of early Egyptian medical practice

SMALLPOX DESCRIBED

The Arab alchemist and physician Muhammad ibn Zakariya ar-Razi (Rhazes) (865–925) created clinical descriptions of smallpox and measles. This enabled doctors to distinguish between the two.

The eruption of smallpox is preceded by a continued fever, pain in the back, itching in the nose and nightmares during sleep. These are the more acute symptoms of its approach together with a noticeable pain in the back accompanied by fever and an itching felt by the patient all over his body. A swelling of the face appears, which comes and goes, and one notices an overall inflammatory colour noticeable as a strong redness on both cheeks and around both eyes. One experiences a heaviness of the whole body and great restlessness, which expresses itself as a lot of stretching and yawning. There is a pain in the throat and chest and one finds it difficult to breath[e] and cough. Additional symptoms are: dryness of breath, thick spittle, hoarseness of the voice, pain and heaviness of the head, restlessness, nausea and anxiety. (Note the difference: restlessness, nausea and anxiety occur more frequently with 'measles' than with smallpox. At the other hand, pain in the back is more apparent with smallpox than with measles.) Altogether one experiences heat over the whole body, one has an inflamed colon and one shows an overall shining redness, with a very pronounced redness of the gums.

The Book of Smallpox and Measles

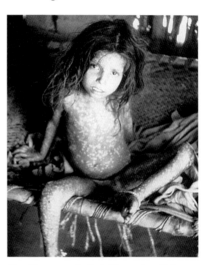

Smallpox pustules look like grains of rice under the skin, and cover the whole body

more than treat the symptoms and hope for the best. Often, there was simply no effective treatment available to combat their condition.

In the hands of the gods

Over the years, physicians have used various methods to reach diagnoses. Some have been magical or superstitious and others have been more or less scientific. Because people believed that gods or evil spirits brought disease, it was natural that they should try supernatural means to cure sickness. That meant either appeasing the malignant influence or driving it away. They also turned to supernatural means to help determine the best course of treatment.

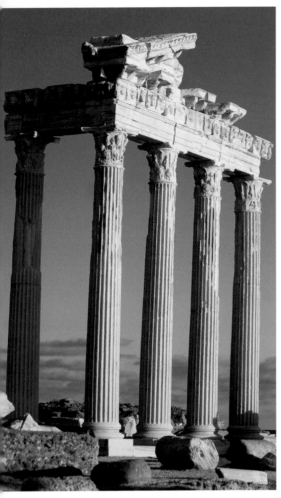

divine healer Imhotep were the venue for temple sleep; in ancient Greece, temples dedicated to Asclepius were favoured. The trance could last up to three days, during which time the attendant priests at the temple or shrine used incantations, rituals and other magical behaviour. Priests were well versed in herbal remedies and dream interpretation; over time the part played by medicinal herbs increased while the magical element declined. Satisfied patients left votive offerings in the form of clay models of the body parts that had been healed and inscriptions detailing the kind of cure that they had received. Temple sleep created many satisfied customers, if we can judge from the massive number of votive parts that have survived: ten cubic metres of them have been excavated from the Asclepieion at Corinth. The Romans adopted temple sleep from the Greeks and built temples to Apollo throughout their empire. The practice is still current in some

The temple of Apollo at Side, Antalya, in Turkey where 'temple sleep' offered the hope of a divine cure to the sick and ailing

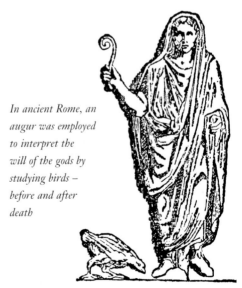

In ancient Rome, an augur was employed to interpret the will of the gods by studying birds – before and after death

The ancient Egyptians and the ancient Greeks often turned to 'temple sleep' in the hope of a divinely-revealed cure. Patients were put into a trance before going to sleep in a special temple, hoping for dreams that would reveal something of the nature of their illness and its appropriate treatment. In Egypt, the temples of the

parts of the Middle East and North Africa.

In addition to the revelations that came from dreams, the ancient Greeks and Romans used augury as a means of obtaining directions from the gods. A patient made a sacrifice – often a bird – and the priest would then read the intestines of the slaughtered creature to find information about the problem and its cure.

Signs and symptoms

As dependence on divine revelation waned, physicians came to rely on more mundane (and reliable) ways of deciding on a course of treatment. While a patient's subjective account of their condition – their symptoms – is useful for a physician, it is not always reliable or even available: patients who are unconscious, or small children, can give no account of their symptoms. So although taking a history is a good start, the signs of disease – the objective evidence measured or observed by an expert – can be more useful to medical investigators.

In ancient Chinese medicine, physicians tried to determine the balance of yin and yang in their patient. Making a diagnosis involved asking detailed questions about the history of the illness, the state of the patient's senses of smell and taste and the nature of their dreams. While the patient talked, the doctor noted the sound of their voice and the colour of their face and tongue. Most importantly, the physician took the patient's pulse at several points on the body using different methods. The same pulse was often taken several times. The book *Meh Ching (Classic of the Pulse)*, written by Wang Shu-ho in the 3rd century AD, explains how the doctor may determine the

> **THE VOCABULARY OF MEDICINE**
> The place where patients lay down at a healing shrine or temple was called a *kline*, which gave us the modern word 'clinic' and the period of treatment was known as 'incubation'. Asclepius, in his semi-divine state, had two daughters named Hygieia (the goddess of health) and Panaceia (the goddess of healing), which gave us the words 'hygiene' and 'panacea' (a cure-all).

nature of the patient's condition, how the illness will progress and even the time at which the patient will recover or die – all deduced from the pulse.

In ancient India, doctors examined patients thoroughly. They palpated them and listened to the heart, lungs and abdomen. If a bone was broken they even listened to the broken ends grinding together, which would hardly have been pleasant for the patient. They also examined the state of the skin and the tongue. In ancient Egypt, doctors assessed patients using a method similar to modern triage. They decided whether a patient could be cured, might improve or would certainly die.

The ancient Greeks, too, used all their senses when trying to assess the state of the patient. At the time of Hippocrates (c.460–375BC), more emphasis was placed on prognosis (determining the outcome of the condition) than on diagnosis (identifying its nature). This makes good sense, since knowing whether the patient would live or die was of more use than identifying a condition for which there was probably no reliable treatment anyway. Hippocrates set great store by uroscopy – examining the urine of the patient – but again he was using it principally as a tool for prognosis. Galen (AD129–c.216) followed suit. More than a thousand years after Hippocrates, Theophilus (fl.7th century AD) initiated uroscopy as a means of diagnosis. His work *De urinis* set the pattern for much of the diagnostic practice of the Middle Ages, and uroscopy remained the principal diagnostic tool until the 18th century. The physician would examine the colour of the urine before smelling it and tasting it. He then looked for deposits and precipitates and carried out simple tests.

For nearly two thousand years, physicians in Europe diagnosed with the intention of identifying the imbalance in the humours that lay at the root of the patient's

The medieval urine wheel linked the colour and properties of a patient's urine to their condition

distress. Their findings would supposedly provide the key to treatment.

The records of the English physician John Symcotts (1592–1662) show how the humours featured in diagnosis. He wrote to one patient:

Your high coloured urine is an apparent sign of inflammation of blood and multitude of choleric humours which... are carried upwards, fixed in the bordering parts of the brain, causing that pain, noise and impostumous matter which you complain of.

The patient's treatment was intended to oppose and correct their condition, so treatment for a wet, cold illness would be designed to provide dry warmth. For

Presentation	Diagnosis	Treatment
Patient is feverish, dry	excess yellow bile	cold baths
Patient is feverish, sweating and flushed	excess of blood	bleeding
Patient is cool, dry, lethargic	excess black bile	build up blood, feed patient red meat, red wine
Patient is cold, wet, sluggish	excess phlegm	induced sneezing, heat, hot foods

Humoral theory and its corresponding treatment dominated western medicine for almost two millennia

example, Symcotts proposed to treat another patient

... first, by a gentle purgative way to abate such serous and waterish humours... In the second place, I should prescribe bleeding... in regard of the hotter temper of your liver, the fountain of redounding choler which, insinuating into the veins, sharpens the blood and humours thereof and causeth by turns that inflammatory humour of your eyelids, mordacity of urine... After this, I shall proceed to things rather of a drying than astringent nature...

It may look like gobbledegook now, but it all seemed to make good sense at the time. The humours formed the basis for diagnosing mental illness, too. One of Symcotts' contemporaries described a patient who was

Very melancholic, delighting in solitariness. He thinketh that he speaketh foolishly and in vain. And imagineth that he is weak and that his legs and body is worn away.

In another case, he clearly thought the patient was a complete lunatic because he noted the signs of the moon beside his account of her case. It was widely believed that lunacy followed the phases of the moon (indeed, the very term 'lunacy' is a derivative of the Latin 'luna' meaning 'moon') and part of the diagnosis of madness involved linking changes in behaviour to the moon's phases.

Tricks and tools of the trade

Modern medicine relies on a battery of tests and a cabinet of tools, ranging from the simplest thermometers and stethoscopes to the most advanced technologies such as MRI (magnetic resonance imaging) scanners and fibre-optic endoscopes. But until the 19th century, doctors had none of these. The earliest diagnostic tools were simple probes and specula (which hold open the mouth, rectum or vagina for inspection of the interior).

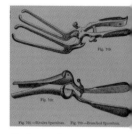

Early specula helped doctors to peer inside patients

For centuries, doctors depended on their powers of observation and their sense of touch. They held a hand to a patient's brow to judge their temperature and they felt the patient's pulse with their fingertips. Until the late 17th century, most clocks had no minute or second hands, so even counting the pulse accurately was difficult – although from the 14th century onwards physicians measuring the pulse rate could use a small hourglass filled with powdered eggshell as a timer. Otherwise, doctors could only compare the patient's pulse with their own, or make subjective judgments about whether it was fast, slow, or uneven.

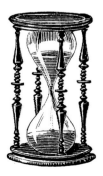

An egg timer gave the doctor a way of counting the pulse over a fixed period of time

91

The body's secret sounds

Early physicians set great store by listening to the sounds within a patient, but for thousands of years they could only do it by putting their ear to the patient's chest or abdomen. Not everyone was comfortable with this. René Théophile Hyacinthe Laënnec hit upon the idea of the stethoscope in 1816 when he felt uneasy about putting his head on the bust of a stout young patient. After creating a decent distance between his ear and the young woman's bosom by using a rolled-up piece of paper, he found that he could hear the sounds in her chest better than ever. He then began to experiment with a simple wooden tube. After several refinements, a stethoscope with two earpieces appeared. In 1850 George Camman produced the precursor of the modern stethoscope, with

René Théophile Hyacinthe Laënnec invented the stethoscope in 1816

two earpieces and a flexible rubber tube replacing the stiff materials used previously. The stethoscope enabled physicians to hear more sounds from the heart and the lungs than ever before and to identify unusual activity more accurately. It increased knowledge about natural and unnatural heart rhythms and the way in which blood moves within the heart. Only by knowing what is normal can a doctor identify and quantify the abnormal.

Pumping blood

Nowadays the stethoscope is commonly used with a sphygmomanometer to measure blood pressure, but blood pressure was not always measured so cleanly. William Harvey

---

THE FIRST STETHOSCOPE

Here Laënnec recalls the time he first thought of using an aid to help him listen to a patient's chest:

I recalled a well-known acoustic phenomenon: namely, if you place your ear against one end of a wooden beam the scratch of a pin at the other extremity is distinctly audible. It occurred to me that this physical property might serve a useful purpose in the case with which I was then dealing. Taking a sheet of paper I rolled it into a very tight roll, one end of which I placed on the precordial region [of the patient's chest], whilst I put my ear to the other. I was both surprised and gratified at being able to hear the beating of the heart with much greater clearness and distinctness than I had ever before by direct application of my ear [to the chest].

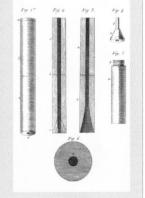

Laënnec's stethoscope, the forerunner to those used by doctors today

Stephen Hales, the first man to measure blood pressure

(1578–1657) noticed that blood spurted from a cut artery with a steady rhythm – it didn't just flow as a spilled liquid would.

The first person to try to measure blood pressure was the English physiologist Stephen Hales. In around 1706 he inserted a brass pipe into an animal's blood vessel and then linked the pipe to a vertical glass tube, using the windpipe of a goose as a flexible connector. He was able to calculate the animal's blood pressure by measuring

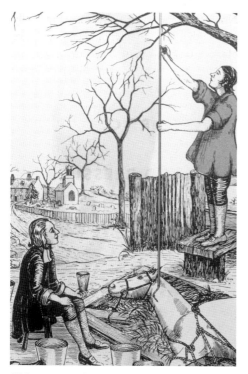

Hales measures the blood pressure of a horse in 1727, using a glass tube

the height reached by the spurting liquid. He obtained his most dramatic result by tying a horse to a door laid on the floor: the horse's blood sprang 9.5 feet (2.9 metres) up the glass tube, which was itself nearly 13 feet (4 metres) tall. Clearly this was not a useful method for measuring the blood pressure of a human patient.

In 1828, the French physician Jean Leonard Marie Poiseuille used a U-shaped mercury-filled tube, calibrated in millimetres, to measure blood pressure, but he still needed to pierce a blood vessel. The first measuring device that did not injure the patient was designed by the German physician Samuel Siegfried von Basch in 1876. This was replaced in 1896 by Italian Scipione Riva-Rocci's sphygmomanometer, which was a close forerunner of the modern device. It had an inflatable cuff and a mercury manometer, which measured the force needed to stop the flow of blood. However, only the systolic pulse (when the heart muscle is contracting) could be measured. The breakthrough came in 1905 when the Russian surgeon Nikolai Korotkov, working in the Imperial Medical Academy in St Petersburg, Russia, used a stethoscope with a sphygmomanometer. Using both together, he could detect a pattern of sounds which start when the pressure exerted by the cuff is equal to the systolic pressure, and stop when it is equal to the diastolic pressure. This led to the current method of recording blood pressure and to blood pressure readings accurate enough to reveal hypertension (chronic high blood pressure). But even when hypertension was diagnosed, doctors had no way of working out what caused it or how to treat it.

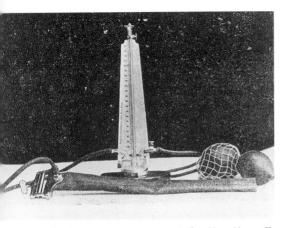

A sphygmomanometer uses an inflatable rubber cuff and a column of liquid against a graduated scale to measure blood pressure

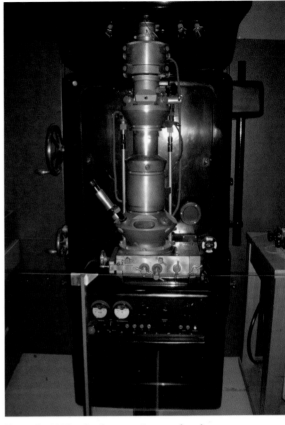

From the 1930s, the electron microscope has shown viruses, bacteria and human cells in great detail, allowing greater scope for analysis and diagnosis

Hot and cold

The other primary diagnostic tool is the clinical thermometer. Galileo invented a crude device for measuring temperature at the end of the 16th century, but it was affected by pressure and it had no scale. Santorio then devised the thermoscope – an early version of the clinical thermometer – in around 1625, but it was difficult to use.

It was not until the early 18th century that the thermometer began to be used in the medical world. An early adopter was Anton De Haen (1704–76), who studied the diurnal changes in healthy subjects and the changes in temperature that accompanied fever. He discovered that the assessment of body temperature was useful in determining the progress of the patient's condition. Even so, the thermometer was not widely adopted. Carl Wunderlich took more than a million temperature readings from over 2,500 patients and then published the results in 1868. His findings indicated a mean normal body temperature of

The Galilean thermometer uses liquid density to measure temperature

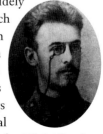

Nikolai Korotkov

36.3 to 37.5 degrees centigrade, and that temperatures higher or lower than this indicated illness. But he took his readings using a thermometer a foot (30.5 cm) long, which was held under the armpit for 20 minutes. The unwieldiness of thermometers meant that they were not widely used until Sir Thomas Clifford Allbutt produced a portable 6-inch (152 mm) thermometer in 1866. Allbutt could read a patient's temperature in just five minutes. By the 1880s, the thermometer had become a standard item in the doctor's medical bag and had taken on a central role in diagnosis.

One of the most important diagnostic tools is not specific to medicine and is not used directly on the patient. The microscope has become an essential

A simple clinical thermometer makes it easy for people to take their own temperature

mainstay of diagnosis. Bacteria, protozoa and parasites can be identified using a microscope and the microscopic examination of cells can reveal cancerous changes and other indications of tissue disease or damage. Family doctors in the second half of the 19th century sometimes viewed samples through microscopes.

They hoped to identify anaemic conditions by examining red blood cells and looked for pus in the urine, which would indicate a urinary tract infection. But, as one American doctor remarked:

BEYOND MERCURY

Although standard mercury thermometers can be very accurate, they have fallen out of use in many developed countries, at least in hospitals. Modern variations include digital thermometers, infrared thermometers that measure the temperature in the ear, and phase-change thermometers. A phase-change thermometer is a plastic strip holding a number of cells (or blisters) which contain chemicals with different melting points mixed in different proportions. When a particular cell reaches a certain temperature, the chemicals melt and the cell changes colour. The patient's temperature is measured by comparing the colour of the cells with a scale on the thermometer.

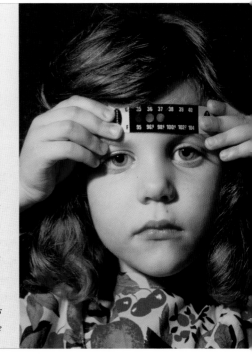

Using a phase-change thermometer such as this one is simple, quick and non-invasive

... [it] will not only assist you in diagnosis, etc., but will also aid you greatly in curing people by heightening their confidence in you and enlisting their co-operation.

Microscopy is now used extensively in hospital laboratories, where diagnoses are made from samples of tissue or fluid, and operating microscopes help surgeons to examine tissue in situ while they are carrying out microsurgery.

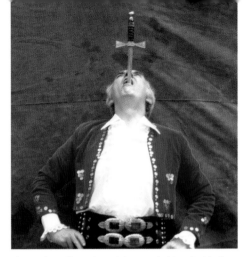

A sword-swallower's training made him the ideal subject of the first endoscopic examination

Looking within

With the advent of anaesthetics, it became theoretically feasible to look inside the body of a living patient. Even so, the risk of infection remained high and surgery was not undertaken lightly. During the 20th century, improvements in antisepsis and the development of antibiotics at last made exploratory surgery worth the gamble and surgeons would, on occasion, open up a patient without knowing what they might find. But even with a reduced risk of

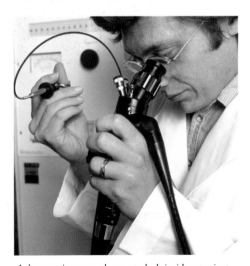

A doctor using an endoscope to look inside a patient

infection, being sliced open is traumatic and uncomfortable and it was not long before better methods were developed.

In 1910, the Swedish surgeon Hans Christian Jacobaeus carried out the first surgical laparoscopic examination. He made a small incision in the patient's abdomen and then inflated the area with air and examined it using an early endoscope called a cystoscope. The modern endoscope is a long flexible tube with a fibre optic light and a camera built into it. It is fed through a small incision or through a natural opening (often the mouth) to reveal the inside of the body. The first endoscopes were just used to investigate natural openings. An early endoscope was found in the ruins of Pompeii, the Roman town that was destroyed by a volcanic eruption in AD79, and a form of endoscope was also used in ancient Greece, according to the Hippocratic texts.

The first modern attempt at endoscopy was made by Philip Bozzini in 1805. He used a tube he called a Lichtleiter to look inside the urinary tract, the rectum and the pharynx. A real breakthrough came in 1868 when for the first time a doctor observed the inside of the stomach of a living subject. Adolph Kussmaul of Germany persuaded a professional sword-swallower to gulp down a straight metal tube, 47 cm (18.5 inches) long and 1.3 cm (0.5 inch) in diameter. This was obviously out of the question for patients who were not trained in sword-swallowing. Rudolph Schindler developed a more useful endoscope in 1932. A series of mirrors inside a flexible tube reflected the image that was illuminated by a light bulb at its end. Then in 1949 a Japanese company first added a camera to an endoscope, which recorded monochrome still images on to physical film. Since then, endoscopes have moved on to using fibre optics, which deliver high definition television images (HDTV) to display screens, and tiny, self-contained capsule endoscopes which travel through the entire gut gathering images. Endoscopes can even incorporate ultrasound in order to obtain images of the layers below the surface of the gastrointestinal tract.

X-RAY VISION

Using rays of energy to reveal what lies

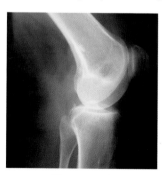

X-rays reveal damage to bones which cannot otherwise be seen

inside a patient is much better than making even a small hole. The first X-ray of the human body was made by Wilhelm Röntgen in 1895 – it shows his wife's hand. X-rays were soon used medically, as a way of revealing broken or diseased bones, and

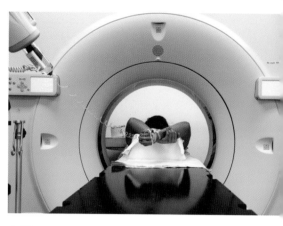

CAT scanners enable doctors to produce computerized 3D images of the inside of a patient's body

quickly became a popular diversion at parties, too.

X-rays show up bones easily, but using them to reveal problems with soft tissues is trickier. The first successful method required the patient to swallow gas-inducing pellets to inflate the stomach, followed by a barium meal (an unpalatable chalky concoction containing barium sulphate, that is opaque to X-rays). The barium sulphate coats the inside surface of the oesophagus and the stomach and any blockages, growths or lesions show up on an X-ray. A similar method using a barium enema shows the lower intestine. Barium meals and enemas have been largely replaced by endoscopy.

A more revolutionary use of X-rays came in 1972 with the invention by Sir Godfrey Newbold Hounsfield of the CT or CAT (computed axial tomography) scanner. Only possible after the invention of computers, the CAT scanner processes multiple X-rays to produce a three-dimensional image of the inside of the body.

FRAU RÖNTGEN'S HAND

In 1895 X-rays were discovered accidentally by Wilhelm Röntgen, professor of physics at the University of Würzburg, Germany. He found that when he sparked the gas in a Crookes tube (an early type of cathode ray tube) a glow appeared on a nearby fluorescent screen. But when he wrapped the tube in cardboard to exclude visible light, the screen still glowed. He then tried thicker materials, including aluminium sheet and lead. When he moved his hand in front of the screen, he was astonished to see an image of the bones in his hands. He used photographic film to make a permanent record of the incredible image, the first ever X-ray. Six weeks later, on 22 December 1895, he made an X-ray image of his wife's hand, which has become the most famous medical image of all time. X-rays were used to examine fractures from January 1896 onwards, the month following his discovery. In 1901 he was awarded the Nobel Prize.

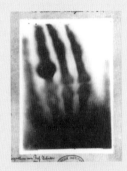

Frau Röntgen's hand, with her wedding ring

It has revolutionized the diagnosis of cancer and other soft-tissue diseases. Hounsfield shared the Nobel Prize for Physiology or Medicine in 1979 with Allan MacLeod Cormack, who developed the mathematics behind the technique.

SOUND AND VISION

Other methods using energy to image the inside of the body include ultrasound, MRI (magnetic resonance imaging) and PET (positron emission tomography). Ultrasound was the earliest of these methods to be used. The Austrian Karl Theodore Dussik published the first paper on using ultrasound in medicine in 1942, after using ultrasound to investigate the brain. In 1950 a Scottish doctor, Ian Donald, developed many more practical applications. Thanks to the work of another Scot, Stuart Campbell, in the 1970s, ultrasound has become widely used as a way of identifying problems in babies developing in the womb. The progress of a normal foetus can also be measured and assessed using ultrasound.

The first successful nuclear magnetic resonance (NMR) experiment was completed in 1946 and medical uses of MRI soon followed. MRI uses a powerful magnetic field to produce and then measure a rotating magnetic field in the hydrogen atoms within the body. In 1971 Raymond Damadian showed that MRI can be used to

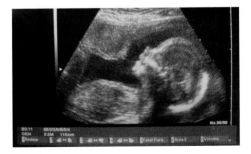

An ultrasound scan reveals a foetus in the womb

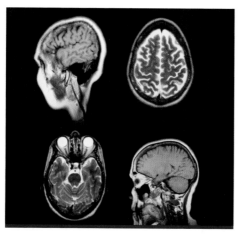

A high-res MRI scan of a brain vasculature, showing a normal brain from all angles

A PET scan uses radioisotopes to show brain activity (left) with normal 'before' images as a control (right)

distinguish between healthy tissue and tumours and in 1977 he demonstrated the first full body scan using MRI. MRI is now used for diagnosing many different medical conditions, including brain problems.

The concept of the PET scan emerged in 1950, but the techniques used in modern scanning were not developed until the late 1970s. A radioisotope with a short half-life is chemically incorporated into a molecule that is used by the body (usually a sugar), and then injected into the subject. The isotope is taken up by the body and becomes part of the body's chemical processes. By measuring the radioactive emissions, the scanner builds up a picture of the inside of the body. PET scans are used to map normal brain and heart function and to diagnose tumours and brain conditions. Because a PET scan shows chemical activity as it happens, it can reveal the parts of the brain that are active at any given moment, so it has greatly increased our knowledge of which areas of the brain perform which functions.

Man and machine

Doctors are now assisted by computers running databases containing thousands of possible conditions and their treatments. Even so, the most important elements in any diagnosis are the doctor and the patient: a stethoscope or an MRI scanner is of no use in the hands of someone without medical knowledge. The renowned Canadian physician Sir William Osler (1849–1919) placed great emphasis on conducting a detailed physical examination and listening to the patient's own account of the condition. One of his many aphorisms was, 'If you listen carefully to the patient they will tell you the diagnosis'. This truth remains central to diagnosis, even with the battery of chemical tests and medical machinery available to the modern hospital.

Wise words: Sir William Osler

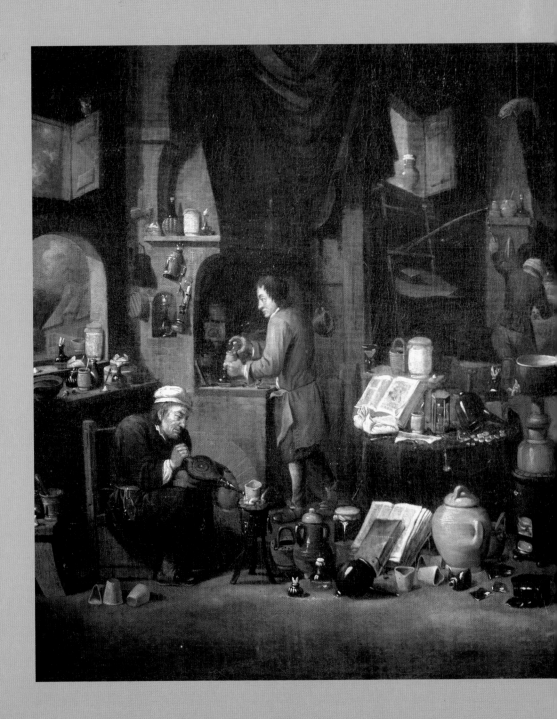

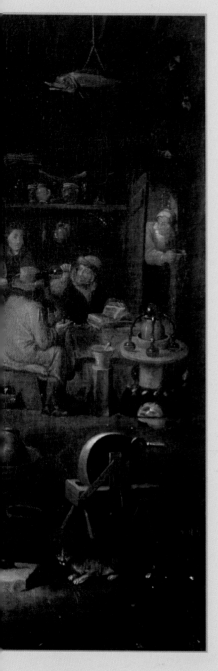

CHAPTER 4

TREATMENT

On a good day, diagnosis leads to a course of treatment that will make the patient well again – or at least make their remaining life more comfortable. But for thousands of years treatment was very much a hit-or-miss affair. Doctors treated symptoms, rather than causes, and hoped for the best. If the patient was lucky the treatment worked, but many people became worse or even died. Just as often, the treatment made little difference one way or the other.

Treatments have ranged from magic spells and incantations, through medicines and potions to rituals and procedures. Medicines have been made from plants, but also from parts of animals, from metals and minerals and even some unlikely, bizarre and downright unpleasant ingredients – such as crushed mummified bodies and body fluids from other sufferers. Procedures have included making people sick, drawing copious quantities of blood from patients who were already ill, and trying to transfer the illness to an inanimate object. There has been no end to the methods desperate patients and their doctors have been willing to try.

A 17th-century doctor's shop offered scores of medicinal concoctions for the sick and infirm in their search for relief

Beyond human powers

If people believe that gods, spirits and magical powers are responsible for illness they will naturally turn to supernatural means in the search for a cure. These expedients range from prayers to spells to self-immolation. It is not only in ancient or undeveloped societies that people have resorted to the paranormal. In the desperation of illness, people will turn to any possible source of succour and hope.

GODS TO THE RESCUE

In ancient Egypt medicine was a strange mixture of myth, superstition and skilled practical treatment. Many Egyptian doctors believed that the remedies for diseases were

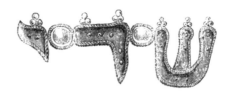

For thousands of years, people have used amulets like this Shaddai charm to ward off illness

revealed by the god Thoth and that these were preserved in secret books in the temples of Sais or Heliopolis. They treated many symptoms with a magical incantation, at least as a first recourse. Incantations are cheap and painless, and were probably the first port of call for patients in many societies. In some cases, no doubt, the illness got better on its own – perhaps the patient's belief in the efficacy of the incantation helped.

As we have seen (see p.88), the practice of 'temple sleep' was common in ancient Greece and Rome. The patient was put to sleep in a special temple in the hope that the gods would communicate a cure in a dream. Temple sleep often produced a prescription, supposedly sent directly from the gods. Fortunately for the physician, the divine intervention meant that he could not be held responsible if the patient did not recover.

Even when illness was accounted for by unbalanced humours or energies, or invisible agents in the air, the belief lingered that an individual could have been singled out by the gods, the spirits or fate to endure ill health. Even today, patients who hold religious beliefs often pray for recovery. Muslims may wear Qur'anic verses as a talisman to help cure specific ills, for instance. This talisman, or charm, is known as a taweez.

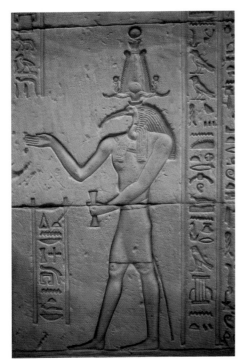

The Egyptian god Thoth was believed to reveal cures for diseases

Thousands of pilgrims of many faiths make their way to religious shrines each year in the hope of a miraculous cure, and some claim that their prayers have been answered. In Christian tradition, some saints are associated with particular diseases. St Valentine is considered the patron saint of people with epilepsy, for instance, while St Roch was rather busier, for he was venerated for curing the plague-stricken. People would go on pilgrimages to shrines associated with the relevant saint, or they might sometimes visit general-purpose shrines. A miraculous spring at Lourdes, France, has been said to cure numerous ailments; each year thousands of pilgrims make their way there in the hope of a cure.

MAGICAL MEANS

The practice of 'conjure' (hoodoo, or folk voodoo) amongst black slaves in America relied on the belief that spells and charms could make people ill, as well as cure them.

In the late 19th century, one victim claimed to have been cured of insanity after a conjure doctor (conjurer) helped her father find an evil charm that was buried near the corner of her house. The charm was a silhouette of the woman that had been cut from black cloth, pierced with pins and hidden in a barrel beneath the soil. When the charm was removed, the woman recovered her sanity. The conjurer also revealed the identity of the person who had supposedly cast the spell. He told the father to inscribe a circle around the house and sprinkle it with an unidentified white powder. Within half an hour, the originator of the curse had visited the house but was unable to cross the magical barrier. For

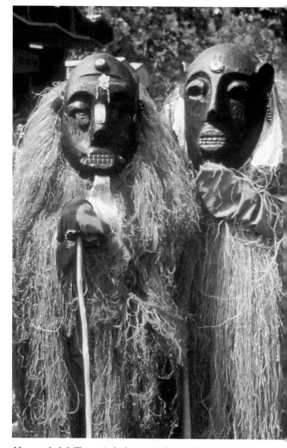

Here to help? Two witch doctors in Lassa, Togo

extra money, conjure doctors would sometimes turn the spell back on the person who had originally cast it. The patient then had the satisfaction of revenge as well as cure. Conjurers would also provide charms and potions to ward off illness. They even claimed the ability to prevent whippings and thrashings, though the slave had to find a way of administering the potion to the slave master for this stratagem to work.

A belief in magical medicine has been shared by people all over the world. In medieval Transylvania, a new mother was

103

required to cut a cockerel or a hen in half (depending on the gender of her child) and then nail the two sections to the doorpost. It was thought that the strength of the bird would pass to the mother, helping her to regain her health.

Even people with access to medical practitioners would sometimes resort to magic. In Europe, poor people, and those in the countryside, often turned to wise women, who combined a scientific or pseudo-scientific knowledge of herbs with superstitious practices and spells in their attempts to heal patients. Writing at the end of the 16th century, the Essex clergyman George Gifford complained that the wise women offering medical services endangered the souls of the faithful:

A man is sick, his sickness doth linger upon him, some do put into his head that he is bewitched, he is counselled to send unto a cunning woman, she says he is forespoken indeed, she prescribes what to use, there must be charms and sorcery used. The party finds ease, he is a glad man... Yet now [he] cannot say that the Lord is [his] health and salvation, but [his] physician is the Devil.

Notice that Gifford did not complain that the medicine of the 'cunning woman' did not work, just that it was ungodly.

Until as recently as 1850 a Welsh cure for epilepsy involved bathing in a magic well and then walking around it three times while reciting the Lord's Prayer. The patient then had to throw money into the well and spend the night beneath the altar of the church with a cockerel or a hen. By morning, the sickness should have passed to the bird, leaving the patient cured. It was a curious mix of local superstition and established religion.

DEAL WITH THE VAMPIRE, DEAL WITH THE DISEASE

In 1883, Mary Brown of Exeter, Rhode Island, died of a mysterious illness (almost certainly TB), followed six months later by her 20-year-old daughter Mary Olive. Nine years later, Mary Olive's 19-year-old sister Mercy fell ill and died of the same illness. Shortly afterwards, their brother Edwin suddenly became frail and sickly.

Convinced that a vampire was causing Edwin's illness, his family and friends exhumed the bodies of Mary, Mary Olive and Mercy. The first two had been reduced to bones, but Mercy's body was preserved. Her teeth and hair seemed to have grown and she had half turned over in her coffin. One of the party cut into her heart and reported that copious quantities of red blood flowed from it. This proved, they thought, that Mercy was the vampire who was draining Edwin's lifeblood. In the hope of vaccinating Edwin against the vampire they cut out Mercy's heart and burnt it, then mixed the ashes into a drink for Edwin. Unsurprisingly, the 'vaccination' was not effective: Edwin died two months later.

Restoring the balance

In both the East and the West, restoring balance in the body was the aim of most therapies. In the East, the balance of yin and yang, and the healthy flow of energy, remained the targets of medical treatment for thousands of years. Chinese physicians saw an imbalance in the body's yin and yang as the cause of all diseases. It was thought that the balance could be restored by using herbal medicines, acupuncture or moxibustion. (Moxibustion involves burning a substance on the body, then pushing the ashes into the blister that forms at the site.)

If the Chinese physician followed the herbal route he would treat a yin condition by using herbs with cold or moist properties, or a salty, sour or bitter taste. A yang condition was believed to respond to herbs with hot or dry properties, or sweet or insipid flavours. Acupuncture or acupressure would be used to block or unblock various energy pathways or cut off pain, thereby allowing the body to relax and heal itself.

Indian medical authorities advised that the whirling energy of the chakras must be kept in good order if physical or mental illness was to be avoided. The chakras could be rebalanced and unblocked by meditation, or by using acupuncture, oils or crystals. In the West, from the time of Hippocrates until the 19th century, doctors sought to balance the four humours as a way of preventing or treating physical and mental illness. Some of the methods used were common to all cultures: bloodletting and the use of therapeutic drugs were at the forefront of the physician's armoury in all parts of the world.

'Bad Blood' and Other Ill Humours

Hippocrates recommended three stages to treatment: advice about diet and lifestyle; treatment with drugs if the first did not work; and surgery as a last resort. His diet and lifestyle advice was directed towards rebalancing the humours. So for an illness that was deemed cold and dry, for example, he would advocate hot drinks and spicy food. If this moderate approach was unproductive, more radical measures followed. Later doctors often missed out the first stage, especially once people began to expect pills and potions (and became reluctant to pay for simple dietary advice).

The Hippocratic model did not always describe the balance of the body with reference to the humours. It could also be

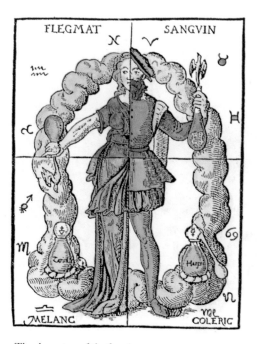

The characters of the four humours

described in terms of the elements (earth, air, fire and water), which were considered the basic building blocks of everything – including the humours. Or doctors might refer to contrasting powers (hot and cold, moist and dry), and even 'fluxes' that could settle in the wrong place in the body. To remove excess moisture, physicians induced sweating; to remove excess bile, they resorted to purging with emetics and laxatives; to remove surplus phlegm, they induced sneezing; to cure someone with too much blood, they bled the patient.

Blood will out

Bleeding as a treatment was not restricted to the cultures that subscribed to the humorist model. The people of ancient Mesopotamia and Egypt used therapeutic bleeding, as did the Mayans and the Aztecs in South America.

Hippocrates had based his confidence in bleeding on menstruation, which he saw as nature's way of ridding women of bad humours. Galen furthered the cause by declaring that while the blood that flowed into the extremities was normally used up, in abnormal circumstances it could build up and stagnate, leading to illness. The way to cure the patient was to remove the stagnant blood by bleeding. Galen also believed that blood was the humour most in need of control. He drew up complex guidelines that described how much blood of which type (arterial or venous) should be drawn for different conditions. He also mapped the blood vessels to various parts of the body and demanded that blood should be taken from specific places. For instance, diseases of the liver should be tackled by bleeding from the vein in the right hand. Arab, and later European, physicians took their cue from Galen and set great store by appropriate bleeding. Superstitious beliefs grew up around bloodletting, too, for both Jewish and Christian practitioners favoured bleeding on particular days and at specific times, in order to obtain the maximum benefit.

SCARIFICATORS, CUPS AND LEECHES

Strictly speaking, bleeding was a surgical procedure. However, it was so widely practised that it had a status of its own. Doctors and barbers, as well as surgeons, carried it out. There were many ways of

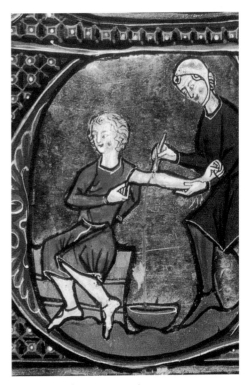

Blood-letting by opening a vein was a common medical practice throughout the world

bleeding a patient. The most obvious technique was to open an artery or a vein ('breathing' it), but later on other methods developed, included scarification, cupping and the use of leeches. While 'breathing' consisted of slitting one of the main veins, often in the arm, scarification was applied to smaller blood vessels. Scarificators have been used throughout history and around the world. The Karaya tribe in Brazil, for example, made a scarificator by using wax to fasten sharp fish teeth to broken pieces of river shell. In 19th-century Europe, scarification boasted a mechanical sophistication that was characteristic of the age. They are rather chilling to modern eyes, having a neat row of blades and a depth adjustment bar to control the severity of the wound. Cupping involved placing heated cups over small incisions in the skin. As the hot air cooled, the reduced pressure in the cup drew blood out of the body and into the cup.

Leeches were used for bleeding by Hippocrates, Galen, Avicenna and the doctors of ancient India, China and Egypt. These natural blood-suckers also became very popular in Europe in the 19th century. During the 1830s, France imported around 40 million leeches a year. The leech produces an anticoagulant that prevents the blood from clotting, thereby allowing the leech to continue sucking until it is completely bloated. It then falls away naturally. Leech saliva also contains an antibiotic and a vasodilator, which encourages blood to flow freely. In most cases, the patient would have been better off without bleeding. However, leeches are again in vogue for treating various

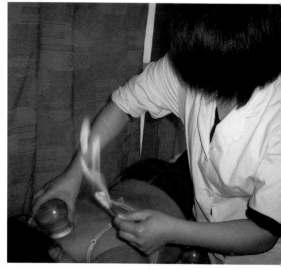

The ancient Chinese procedure of cupping is still practised today. It is used to treat a wide spectrum of diseases and disorders

conditions in which thinning the blood is useful, including some heart disease, arthritis, rheumatism, varicose veins and other types of thrombosis. Modern hospitals use leeches bred in sterile conditions and discard them after a single use to prevent infection.

Bleeding was used as a treatment in the most unlikely circumstances. Often, an injury that produced bleeding was itself treated with further bleeding. It is hard to see the logic in this. As might be expected, there were occasional mishaps. In 1799 George Washington, the first president of America, died after his doctors removed a staggering five pints of blood from him in a single day, while trying to treat a severe throat condition. The jury is still out on whether it was the bleeding that killed him, but it can't have helped. The 17th-century English physician John Symcotts recalled that his father suffered gout so severely that 'in three days it corrupted so his foot to the bone that daily flesh deaded and putrified parts of bones were taken out'. Symcotts advised 'bleeding and purging above 40 times in less than seven weeks space' even though his father was all of 77 years old. Bleeding could be used as a prophylactic, too: frequent bleeding was considered good for the health and it was a treatment offered routinely by barbers. Monks were obliged by religious edict to be bled at regular intervals, so the fortunate barbers who visited the monasteries to carry out the task were assured of a guaranteed income.

Purging

Apart from bleeding, physicians used drugs to encourage patients to vomit, urinate or defecate in order to purge themselves. As with bleeding, there was often no sound reason why the 'cure' should have any beneficial effect, but doctors sometimes hit upon something that worked. For instance, it was considered that syphilis required purging and abstention from sex. Although the latter is a wise precaution, because it prevents the spread of the disease, the physicians of the 15th and 16th centuries simply thought that sex was a drain on the body's energy and so would be detrimental to the patient. The purging component of the treatment for syphilis came in the form of baths or the administration of mercury. In 1502 Jacob Carpensic became the first physician to prescribe mercury for syphilis. The treatment was afterwards widely promoted by Paracelsus (who ensured its universal adoption). Mercury was

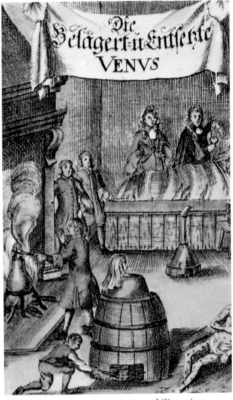

Using mercury vapours to treat syphilis patients

administered orally, painted on to lesions, used in plasters or applied by fumigation. This last method required the patient to be locked in a box in which mercury was heated until it vaporized. Mercury plasters, paints and fumigation induced sweating while ingesting mercury caused spitting. Mercury did produce a beneficial effect but it was not brought about by the spitting and the sweating. Instead, the administration of mercury killed the syphilis spirochetes (the long, coiled, spring-like bacteria that cause syphilis). The medical world had struck lucky. However, because mercury was usually administered in the final stages of

SYPHILIS

Syphilis hit Europe with a vengeance in the 1490s, when it was brought back from South America by explorers. By 1497 it had spread throughout France, and the rest of Europe followed within a decade. The disease has three stages. A chancre (sore) appears at the site of infection (usually the penis) within 2 to 4 weeks of contact with the disease. If this is untreated it heals naturally in 3 to 8 weeks. After a further 6 to 8 weeks the disease progresses to the next stage. The patient feels tired and may develop headaches, fever, swollen glands and a sore throat. There might be weight loss, hair loss and a skin rash. These symptoms can last from 3 to 6 months, coming and going apparently at random. After this, the disease goes into a latent stage, when there are no symptoms. This can last for a considerable time – even the rest of the patient's life. Between 50 per cent and 70 per cent of syphilis patients never progress to the final stage. This is fortunate, because it is deeply unpleasant. The spirochete embeds itself thoroughly into the tissues during the latency period and the final stages of syphilis are characterized by lesions on the skin, bones

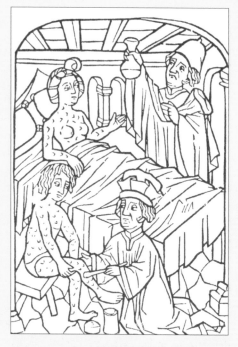

Applying mercury to syphilis lesions was effective, but mercury vapour is highly toxic

and vital organs. The tissues all decay as they are slowly eaten away by the disease. If syphilis affects the brain (neurosyphilis) the patient suffers paralysis and madness.

syphilis, it was rarely possible to administer enough mercury to defeat the disease without killing the patient by mercury poisoning.

Nature's pharmacopoeia

Most of the methods used for inducing purging involved herbal or other medicines that acted as laxatives or emetics. Many cultures have left records of the medicinal use of plants and animals which reveals that humankind has turned to the natural world for medicine since prehistoric times. Susruta lists 760 medicinal plants that were used in ancient India, including cannabis and deadly nightshade. The ancient Egyptians used remedies of both plant and animal origin, which are listed in the medical papyri. They include the expected opium and hemlock, but also the more

THE SEE-THROUGH DOCTOR

The emperor Shen Nung, who is said to have written the first Chinese pharmacopoeia, is still worshipped as the patron god of the Chinese drugs guilds. He is reputed to have tried all of the 365 medicines he lists on himself before giving them to patients. It does not add credibility to the tale, but Shen Nung was said to have been transparent, so that he could easily see the effects of the drugs he tested.

unusual fried mouse and hippopotamus fat. Sumerian clay tablets from more than 4,000 years ago list herbal prescriptions and also describe the medicinal use of animal parts and excreta, as well as various minerals. Traditional Chinese medicine made extensive use of herbal remedies and oils; a manuscript called *Recipes for Fifty-two Ailments* was found in a tomb sealed in 168BC. *The Divine Farmer's Herb-Root Classic*, said to have been written by the legendary emperor Shen Nung some 5,000 years ago, is the earliest Chinese pharmacopoeia: the oldest copies date from the Western Han Dynasty (206BC–AD9). It includes 365 medicines derived from plants, animals and minerals. In the West, the Greeks and then the Romans collected an extensive pharmacopoeia, which was taken over and greatly augmented by the Arab medical scientists.

No doubt the medicinal use of herbs and plants began with trial and error, but some proved effective and were added to the medicine chest, where they stayed for millennia. Many modern medicines are based on these ancient folk remedies. Hippocrates advised his followers to chew the leaves of the willow tree as a way of alleviating pain and the Chinese used willow bark to control fever. Willow bark was also widely used in 18th-century Europe, where it was used to treat fever, inflammation and pain. Modern medicine still uses an active ingredient of willow, acetylsalicylic acid. A crude form of acetylsalicylic acid was first synthesized by the French chemist Charles Frédéric Gerhardt in 1853. After others had refined the process, Friedrich Bayer & Company manufactured and sold it, under the name Aspirin, in 1899. It quickly became popular and its success was completely assured after its use in the flu pandemic of 1918.

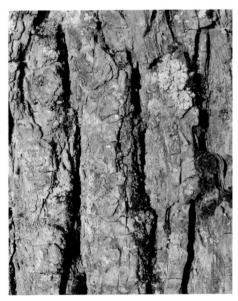

The medicinal use of willow bark may strike us as being rather primitive, but it is from this ingredient that we manufacture aspirin today

FRIAR LAWRENCE'S HERB GARDEN

In Shakespeare's *Romeo and Juliet*, Friar Lawrence explains that plants and stones have been placed on earth for a purpose. Although they all have their medicinal uses he warns that they must be used appropriately, because plants can poison as well as cure.

And from her womb children of divers kind
We sucking on her natural bosom find;
Many for many virtues excellent,
None but for some, and yet all different.
O, mickle is the powerful grace that lies
In plants, herbs, stones, and their true qualities:
For naught so vile that on the earth doth live
But to the earth some special good doth give;
Nor aught so good but, strain'd from that fair use,
Revolts from true birth, stumbling on abuse:
Virtue itself turns vice, being misapplied;
And vice sometimes by action dignified.
Within the infant rind of this small flower
Poison hath residence, and medicine power:
For this, being smelt, with that part cheers each part;
Being tasted, slays all senses with the heart.

Act II, Scene iii

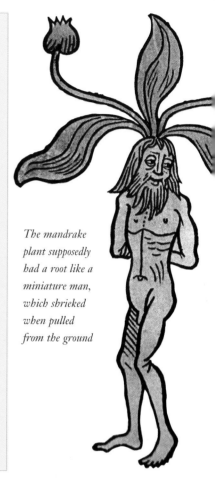

The mandrake plant supposedly had a root like a miniature man, which shrieked when pulled from the ground

One of the most important early modern discoveries of a plant-based drug is quinine, which is effective against malaria. Quinine is extracted from the bark of the cinchona tree, which grows in the Andes. It was discovered by Spanish explorers and conquerors – the very people who carried malaria to South America. In the 1630s, the monk Antonio de la Calancha wrote of the discovery:

A tree grows which they call 'the fever tree' in the country of Loxa, whose bark, of the colour of cinnamon, made into powder amounting to the weight of two small silver coins and given as a beverage, cures the fevers and tertiana [malaria]; it has produced miraculous results in Lima.

It is not clear now whether the drug was known to the indigenous South Americans before the Spanish arrived. Cinchona was not listed in the Inca pharmacopoeia, but the local people could well have discovered the cure in the interval between the arrival of malaria and the Spaniards' discovery of

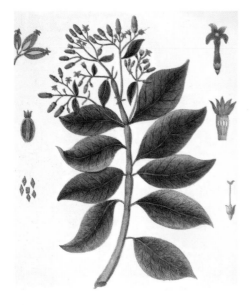

Quinine, the drug used to treat malaria, is extracted from the plant cinchona

Many medical recipes require that medicinal plants should be picked at a certain time of day, often at dawn or dusk. Galen, for example, suggested that some herbs should be gathered before sunrise. This might look like pure superstition but in fact the concentration of alkaloids in many plants varies according to the diurnal cycle of night and day, so there is a sound basis for the practice.

Superstitious or religious belief played a part in the selection of medicinal plants. In the European Middle Ages, Christians believed that God had placed plants and animals on earth to serve humankind and that the cures for all ills could be found once the secrets of creation had been uncovered. It was thought that the form of an object could provide clues – so walnuts, which look similar in structure to the brain, might be good for that organ, or for head

the cinchona tree. The Spanish were happy to use the remedies of the Incas: Francisco Pizarro's soldiers preferred treatment from native healers to the medicine of their own doctors.

In Europe, the Jesuits promoted cinchona and it soon became known as Jesuit's Bark. But the adoption of cinchona bark was hindered by two factors. Firstly, it was widely used for all fevers even though it was only effective against malaria, so its reputation was damaged. Secondly, it was promoted by the Catholic Church. Non-Catholic countries were reluctant to adopt a drug that was advocated by the Vatican. Even so, quinine eventually became the principal malaria treatment. Without it, the British and the Dutch would have taken much longer to colonize India.

A SECRET AND A SCAM

In the late 17th century, Englishman Robert Talbor claimed to have discovered a secret remedy for malaria. At the same time he warned people against the use of Jesuit's Bark. Britain was a Protestant country and would not accept a Catholic remedy anyway. He successfully cured Charles II of malaria and was then sent to France to treat the French royal family. Louis XIV was allowed to buy the recipe on condition that it was not read until after Talbor's death. When Talbor died it was revealed that the secret medicine was, after all, cinchona.

'ALL THE DROWSY SYRUPS OF THE WORLD'

Not poppy, nor mandragora,
Nor all the drowsy syrups of the world,
Shall ever medicine thee to that sweet sleep...
Othello (William Shakespeare), Act III, Scene iii

Sleeping draughts have been prepared throughout history and some of the ingredients are still used. Poppy, in the form of opium, has been used since Neolithic times as a narcotic and painkiller. It is mentioned in the Ebers Papyrus (c.1500BC) and it was used by the Sumerians, Egyptians, Minoans, Greeks, Romans and Persians. Ancient physicians such as Dioscorides, Galen and Avicenna have made reference to it and it provided pain relief in battle until the American Civil War. Morphine, which is administered to current-day battle casualties, is still a derivative of opium.

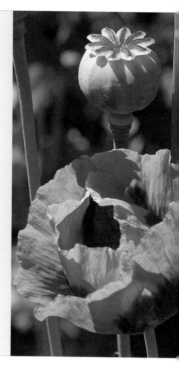

Opium has been obtained from poppies for millennia

ailments in general. In Chinese medicine, too, walnuts were considered good for the brain.

ANIMAL, VEGETABLE OR MINERAL?

Not all medicines are derived from plants. Physicians have often used animals or animal products. The Roman writer Pliny the Elder advised that stewing and eating a red cockerel would protect the consumer against wild beasts while giving him strength. In the Middle

A walnut bears an uncanny resemblance to the human brain, so was often considered a good treatment for the head

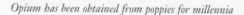

Ages 'cock ale' – made from a boiled cockerel and strong ale – was again supposed to make people strong. Honey has been used for centuries to dress wounds, because it has antiseptic properties. Milk and meat have also been applied to injuries and lesions; the ancient Egyptians tied fresh meat over a crocodile bite, for instance. While animal-based remedies often look more like superstitious magic than real medicine, some would have had a beneficial effect. In ancient China, Shen Nung advised feeding thyroid glands from sheep to children suffering from cretinism. As the condition is a form of hypothyroidism, the treatment could well have helped. Ancient Sumerian doctors prescribed liver for night blindness, and liver is rich in Vitamin A. It is now known that Vitamin A deficiency is a cause of night blindness.

Chemicals and minerals have been used as medicines, too, since the earliest times. The ancient Egyptians used ground up lapis lazuli in some of their treatments, and both gold and pearls were also widely used.

The 16th-century Swiss doctor known as Paracelsus was a pioneering proponent of the benefits of metals and minerals in medicine. Trained in alchemy, he had an extensive knowledge of chemistry which he brought to bear on his medical practice. The most widely used chemical remedy was undoubtedly mercury, which was used to treat syphilis (see p.108). Paracelsus was not the first physician to use mercury, but he became an enthusiastic promoter of the element when he tested it side by side with guaiac, the other commonly used treatment of the time. Made with the bark of the guaiacum tree, guaiac proved to be ineffective.

Gold was used medicinally in ancient Egypt, India and China. The Chinese administered it as a

The unfortunate cockerel has featured as a recipe in medicinal concoctions since at least Roman times

> **PASSING THE BUCK**
>
> Animals did not have to be minced up and consumed to be used medicinally, but any form of medicinal use was rarely a happy experience for the selected creature. Some cures aimed to shift an affliction from a human patient to an animal, others were directed at transferring power from an animal to a person. A cure for warts, recorded in Europe in around 1250, entailed cutting off the head of an eel, rubbing it on the warts and then burying the head. The warts were supposed to heal when the head rotted. An ancient Egyptian cure for blindness was a mixture of mashed pig's eyes, honey and red ochre, which was poured into the ear of the patient. It was thought that the benefit of sight would then pass from the pig to the patient.

treatment for smallpox and measles, for example. Yet the therapeutic use of gold was not confined to the ancients. The fact that gold is not reactive has made it useful in implants, and gold compounds have been used since 1929 in the treatment of rheumatoid arthritis. More unusually, gold is used in the treatment of lagophthalmos, a condition that makes it impossible for sufferers to close their eyes completely. Small gold weights are implanted in the upper eyelid to

PARACELSUS (1493–1541)

Theophrastus Bombastus von Hohenheim was the son of a doctor. He was born in Einsiedeln, Switzerland, but his family moved to the Austrian Tyrol when he was nine. In Austria, he learned about minerals and the secrets of alchemy and astrology. He then travelled extensively as an itinerant physician, working for a time as an army surgeon for the Dutch and the Venetians. In 1526 he healed two famous patients: the printer Frobenius and the philosopher Erasmus. Soon afterwards he was offered a university position in Basle. Although his practice was excellent and his knowledge was intimidating, Paracelsus did not endear himself to the university. He insisted on teaching in German instead of Latin, he began his lectures by burning the works of Galen, and he had no respect for any of the classical authorities except Hippocrates. Furthermore, he accused his colleagues of ignorance and promoting falsehoods. After two years Paracelsus had to leave the university and return to working as a travelling physician. He wrote extensively, introducing important chemical cures into the pharmacopoeia. His enthusiasm for chemistry held Paracelsus back in one important way: he replaced the established humoral theory with his own system of chemical balance. He taught that the human body was composed of three principles, one producing combustibility (sulphur), one liquidity (mercury) and one solidity (salt). An imbalance of these was, he argued, the cause of illness, so restoring the balance by administering the necessary principle would restore health.

Paracelsus soon gained himself a reputation for arrogance

make them heavier. In India, gold is a component of Ayurvedic medicine: when mixed with a herbal ash it is used as a rejuvenator. Several tonnes of gold are consumed each year in this way.

Pearls were used as a medicine in ancient India and China, Tibet and Europe. In China, powdered pearl was ingested in order to detoxify the system, clean the liver, reduce stress or treat a sore throat. It was also applied externally to cuts, sores and burns. In medieval and Renaissance Europe, pearls were used to treat melancholy, palpitations, epilepsy, ulcers, cancer, degeneration in old age, poisoning and plague. Indeed, according to one enthusiast – Anselmus de Boot, the physician to Rudolph II in the 17th century – *aqua perlata* is 'most excellent for restoring the strength and almost for resuscitating the dead'.

CURIOUSER AND CURIOUSER

The more bizarre, outlandish and extravagant the ingredients of a cure, the more it was believed to be effective –

especially if it was also very expensive, like the cures made with gold or pearls. Fantastic concoctions, which seem to have contained as many ingredients as possible, have always been popular. As late as the 17th century, doctors prescribed 'gelly of viper's flesh, broken red coral, sweet almonds, and fresh flowers of blind nettles' as treatment for diabetes. Other European medicines required even more eccentric ingredients, such as iron filings from the fetters of condemned prisoners and – even more difficult to come by – stones from the stomachs of legendary animals. In Chinese medicine, the importance of animal products has pushed some species to the brink of extinction.

The most sought-after cure for plague was the fabled theriac. According to legend, it was first made by King Mithridates VI of Pontus (northern Turkey) in the 1st century BC. He is said to have experimented with poisons and their antidotes, using his prisoners as guinea pigs, and to have found remedies to all known poisons. He mixed all of his antidotes together, adding honey to make the concoction taste better. The result was a general cure-all called Mithridatum; it contained around 50 different ingredients. Mithridates took it each day, because he had a terror of being poisoned. It apparently worked, because he lived to a ripe old age, and when he was defeated by the Roman general Pompey and tried to poison himself, the deadly dose had no effect on him – he had built up an immunity with his repeated small doses.

After the Romans adopted Mithridatum they improved the recipe, taking the ingredient count up to 64. It now included

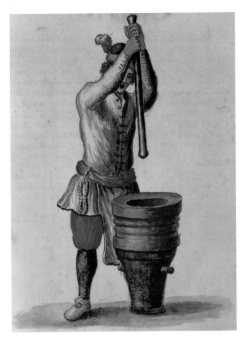

Pounding the ingredients: using some elbow grease has been essential in medicine-making for centuries

roasted and fermented mashed viper flesh, one of the most enduring components. Theriac was taken to China and India, where it also became popular. In Europe, it became such an Italian speciality that the English knew it as Venice treacle. The ingredients, including the ubiquitous viper's flesh and opium, were prepared, matured and mixed with honey. Theriac was aged for at least a year and preferably several years. Ritual and legislation surrounded its production and all the ingredients had to be available for official inspection before work began. The preparation of the mixture became something of a ceremony, which could only be carried out by approved manufacturers. As a result, the finished product was very expensive, so it was only

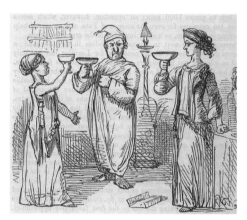

Mithridates' cure-all, a blend of 50 or so ingredients, was used for nearly 2,000 years

available to the rich. Theriac could be made into a syrup, applied as a powder or even eaten in chunks, and it was reputed to cure almost any ailment, including bubonic plague. The recipe was made public by the French apothecary Moyse Charas in 1668, thereby ending the Venetian monopoly on manufacture.

Galen's espousal of theriac no doubt contributed to its enduring popularity, but a London doctor, William Heberden, wrote in 1745 that it offered no benefits besides sweating. As a result, theriac fell out of favour in England, though records show that it was still available in France in 1884. Modern researchers suspect that it might have had some beneficial effects: it contains various strong anti-inflammatory drugs and the opium would have reduced patients' pain and helped to reduce the fever, cough and diarrhoea of the plague.

DAYS OF THE DEAD

One of the most prized ingredients in European medicine was derived from human remains. Mummy, or mumia – an extract of mummified corpses dug from ancient Egyptian tombs – was considered a powerful remedy for many different conditions. It was recommended by Paracelsus, although it was derided by the French surgeon Ambroise Paré (1510–90). Nevertheless, it was hugely popular in Europe from the 12th to the 18th centuries. It was so sought after that unscrupulous traders soon created a trade in fake mumia. They collected dead bodies, stuffed them with bitumen, bandaged them and left them to dry in the sun. A Jewish trader at Alexandria explained the process to Guy de la Fontaine in 1564, adding that he neither knew nor cared whether the victims had died of dangerous diseases such as smallpox or plague.

Skull moss was a useful ingredient that could be acquired without a trip to Egypt. It is a type of moss that grows on human bones. Like mumia, it was believed to contain the life force of the corpse. The skull of a hanged criminal produced particularly valuable skull moss because the spirit was thought to remain trapped in the skull for seven years. The skull had to lie unburied so that the moss could grow. Ireland was considered a good source of skull moss, because criminals were left hanging on the gibbet for a long while.

But there was more to corpse medicine than mummified remains and skull moss. Medicines have been derived from parts of recently dead bodies from the earliest times. The Ebers Papyrus (c.1500BC) reveals that in ancient Egypt a human brain was used to make a medicine for a damaged eye. Half of the brain was added to honey to make an

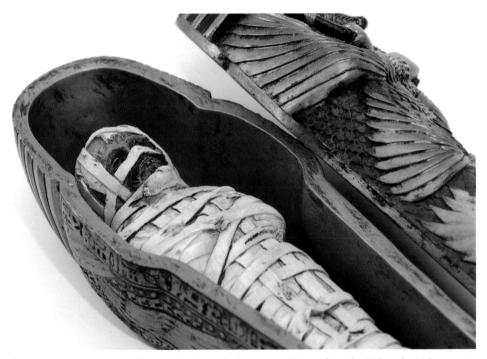

Egyptian mummies were considered a valuable medical resource in Europe from the 12th to the 18th centuries

ointment to apply in the morning and the other half was dried and crushed to make a powder for evening application. In the 1st century AD Celsus recorded that epilepsy had been cured by sufferers drinking hot blood from a newly-slain gladiator, while in the 16th century Paracelsus also extolled the virtues of blood. The blood of a red-haired young man who had suffered a violent death was, he said, the most beneficial. Paracelsus also used a recipe that called for three human skulls distilled with musk, castoreum (a secretion exuded by beavers) and honey. Liquor of pearls and vitriol were sometimes added.

Others followed Paracelsus' theory that the bodies of people who had died quickly, preferably violently, were a particularly

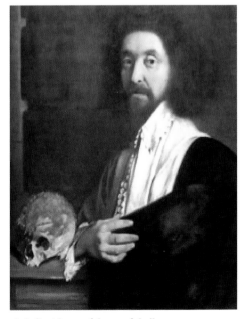

A skull with a useful crop of skull moss

GODDARD'S DROPS, OR SPIRIT OF SKULL

During the 17th century, a Dr Goddard made a concoction from human bones and skulls that he called Goddard's Drops. He dried the bones, distilled them in a retort and then set the distillate aside for three months before heating it for 14 days. He separated the oily layer and added spirit of nitre to create 'a medicine beyond all comparison exceeding the other tenfold in worth and efficacy'. The drops were recommended for epilepsy. Goddard sold the recipe to King Charles II for £6,000 and the king apparently then made the medicine himself in his own laboratory.

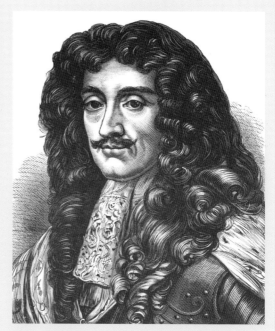

King Charles II was a devotee of Goddard's Drops

valuable source of medicine. People who had bled to death, however, had lost their vital spirits and so were of little or no use. In 18th-century France, human fat was a favoured treatment. It was used as a cure for rheumatism, for instance. According to Pierre Pomet's *A Compleat History of Druggs* (1712), human fat was a perquisite of the public executioner who sold it on the open market in Paris to physicians and apothecaries. And right up until the 19th century epilepsy sufferers crowded around the scaffold on the Danish islands of Amak and Moen, hoping to catch the blood of beheaded criminals in cups.

Before we dismiss the medicinal use of 'homo' (as it was called) as barbaric and unenlightened, it is worth pausing to consider that modern medicine embraces blood and bone marrow transfusions from the living, organ transplants from the dead, and stem cells from the unborn.

WASTE NOT, WANT NOT

Marginally less repellent than medicines made from corpses were the many remedies and ointments made from tissue that could be collected from the living. These included nail parings (an emetic if steeped in wine, unsurprisingly), earwax (useful when applied to scorpion stings), sweat (used against tuberculosis), dried menstrual blood (for the stone and epilepsy), urine (for gout and many other conditions), human excrement (taken by mouth for epilepsy and quinsy, or applied to wounds), fresh blood

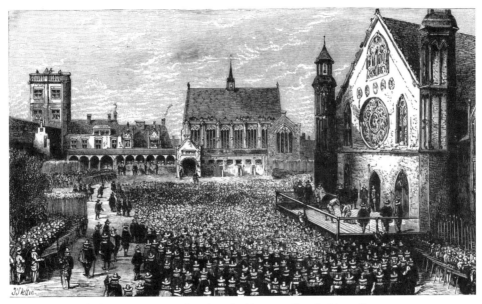

An execution was both an exciting spectacle and a valuable source of medical ingredients

(sometimes sucked from the young by the old in the hope of rejuvenation) and the umbilical cord and the placenta (for epilepsy and, according to Robert James' *Pharmacopoeia universalis* of 1747, 'for destroying noxious vermin').

From apothecaries to pharmacists

Early western pharmacology rests on the work of the Greek physician Dioscorides (c.AD40–c.90), who was one of the greatest army surgeons under the Roman emperor Nero. In *De materia medica* he collected together all of the pharmacological knowledge of the time. Its five volumes dealt with the medicinal uses of herbs, ointments and oils; animal products; plants and roots; wine; and minerals. The text was a principal source of reference that remained in use until the Renaissance.

> **A USEFUL RECIPE**
>
> In *Magia Naturalis* (1558), Giovanni Battista della Porta recorded a prescription for a salve to heal wounds from weapons, given by Paracelsus to the Emperor Maximilian. The weapon that inflicted the wound was to be left lying in the ointment – the ointment was not to be applied to the wound itself.
>
> *Two ounces of skull moss; two ounces of human flesh; half an ounce of mummy; half an ounce of human blood; one ounce of each of linseed oil, turpentine and Armenian bole; pound all the ingredients together in a mortar.*
>
> Book VIII, chapter xii

Initially, physicians administered plant material in its whole form, or made it into a paste, a powder or an infusion that could be ingested, inhaled or applied externally. The Arab scholars, with their advanced development of chemistry, were the first to extract 'simples' or effective substances from their natural sources. Avicenna pioneered the use of distillation and sublimation to extract medicinal ingredients. The Arabs also began to mix compound drugs. The first apothecaries' shops opened in Baghdad in 754 and they first appeared in Europe in the 12th century. In medieval Europe, apothecaries sold and dispensed medicines to patients and to medical professionals. With the further development of chemistry in the 19th century, modern pharmacology began. Chemists extracted the active ingredients that were described in *De materia medica* and made pure preparations of them. Often dissolved in alcohol or water, these substances were administered in carefully measured doses. Controlled clinical trials became a standard means of testing and verifying treatments. Over the last century and a half, biochemists have managed to extract useful, pure forms of drugs from many plants. Some of these drugs no longer have to be extracted from plants but can be synthesized entirely in the laboratory.

In the present century microbes in the soil and fungi have proved to be as valuable as plants, providing powerful antibiotics. Antibiotics and retroviral drugs do more than just treat the symptoms, as many early medicines did; instead, they destroy the agents responsible for causing the disease.

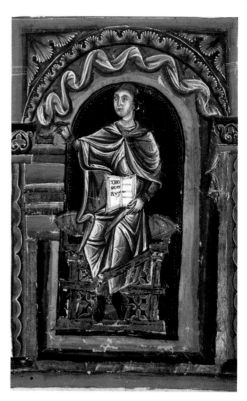

Dioscorides, whose book De materia medica *was the precursor to all modern pharmacopoeias*

Alexander Fleming discovered penicillin, the first antibiotic, in 1928, but he could not produce it in a useful form, so it did not go into large-scale production until the 1940s. The first antibiotics to be used in large quantities were the sulphonamide-based drugs (or sulpha drugs), beginning with Prontosil, which was originally used in the dyeing industry. Its antibacterial nature was discovered by the German chemist Gerhard Domagk in 1935. (Domagk was awarded a Nobel Prize in 1939 for his work on antibiotics, but he was unable to accept it because Hitler had fallen out with the Nobel Committee.)

Many new classes of antibiotics were discovered in the 1940s, 1950s and 1960s and it looked for a while as though humankind would defeat bacterial infection once and for all. But it was not to be. Bacteria evolve quickly and many have already developed forms that are immune to the antibiotics with which we combat them.

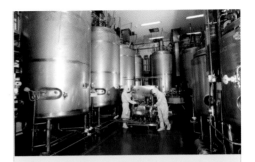

PENICILLIN

Penicillin is an antibiotic prepared from a fungus, *Penicillium notatum*. It was discovered by the Scot Alexander Fleming in 1928, while he was growing *Staphylococcus* bacterial specimens on an agar plate at St Mary's Hospital in Paddington, London. When the plate accidentally became contaminated with the *Penicillium* fungus, Fleming noticed that the *Staphylococcus* bacteria died in circles around the areas of contamination. His work was continued by Howard Florey and Ernst Chain at Oxford and penicillin was isolated in 1940. Soon, it was being produced in vast quantities in the United States. Its use greatly helped to reduce the impact of injury on the Allied forces in the Second World War. Fleming, Florey and Chain shared the Nobel Prize in 1945 for their work on antibiotics.

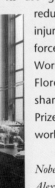

Nobel Prize winner Alexander Fleming, working in his laboratory

MAKING MICROBES WORK

Diabetes sufferers are unable to produce the hormone insulin naturally, so they need to take it as an injection. At one time insulin was harvested from pigs, but in 1977 it became the first hormone to be produced artificially by bacteria. The bacterium that manufactures insulin has been genetically engineered by splicing the gene that is responsible for making insulin into the bacterium. The bacteria are grown in huge vats of nutrients, where they reproduce themselves and produce large quantities of insulin.

The Standing Medical Advisory Committee reported that

In the closing years of the century, there is an uneasy sense that micro-organisms are 'getting ahead' and that therapeutic options are narrowing.

Today, some diseases that could previously be treated with antibiotics are completely resistant and others must be tackled with a potent cocktail of two or more antibiotics. New strains of bacteria such as MRSA (methicillin-resistant *Staphylococcus aureus*), which first appeared

CHEMICALS AGAINST CANCER

The earliest written mention of cancer occurs in the Ebers Papyrus (c.1500BC), which describes breast cancer and goes on to state that the condition is effectively untreatable. It remained so for millennia and it is still one of the greatest challenges facing medical science. For years, the only treatment for cancer was surgery, but from the early 20th century onwards X-rays have been used to deliver radiation therapy.

The first chemical treatments for cancer appeared during the Second World War when the United States Army was investigating chemical weapons. Researchers discovered quite by accident that a compound called 'nitrogen mustard' helps to treat lymphoma (a cancer of the lymph nodes). It became the first in a line of chemical agents that were used to kill rapidly reproducing cancer cells by damaging their DNA. Soon after, American Sidney Farber showed that the drug Aminopterin (related to the vitamin folic acid) stopped the progress of leukaemia in children by blocking DNA replication. A modern cancer drug, methotrexate, was developed from it. In 1956 it was used to cure a rare cancer called choriocarcinoma, so beginning the era of chemotherapy in cancer treatment.

New research into chemotherapy is directed towards reducing the side effects of strong chemotherapy drugs by targeted delivery – that is, taking the drug directly to the site of the cancer in order to reduce damage to other tissue. Methods include packaging the chemical inside liposomes (tiny bubbles made of the same substance as cell membranes) to help them penetrate the cancer cells

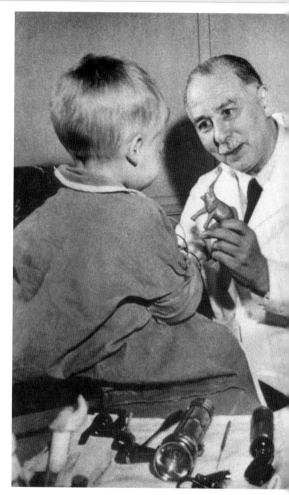

Sidney Farber with a young patient. He was the first doctor to achieve remission in childhood leukaemia using chemotherapy

selectively; using monoclonal antibodies to bind the drugs to the surface of tumour cells; and even using nanorobotic technologies and microscopic magnetic particles to guide the drugs to the cancer site.

in 1961, can be extremely difficult to treat.

As knowledge of chemistry progressed in the second half of the 20th century, it became possible to design drugs 'from the ground up', as it were. By working out the required chemical action at a molecular level, bioengineers can build a molecule to carry out the necessary function. It may interrupt a chemical pathway or bind to the surface of another molecule, for example. Using the 'lock and key' analogy employed by Emil Fischer and Paul Ehrlich over a hundred years ago, one molecule may bind to a position on another (typically a protein) and either perform a function itself or prevent another molecule from occupying that position (and so prevent its function). Biomolecules are modelled using advanced computer technology and then produced in the laboratory. Herceptin, a drug to combat breast cancer, was approved for use in 1998, making it the first bioengineered drug to gain FDA approval.

Leaving well alone

Doctors have often been most successful when they have done least. The body is generally quite good at looking after itself and many conditions will run their course and disappear if over-rigorous interventions do not make matters worse. Hippocrates owed much of his success and fame to what he did not do rather than to what he actually did. His first line of attack in any new case was to advocate a treatment regime that involved adjusting the patient's diet and lifestyle. Nutritious food, exercise and rest in sensible measure will rarely make a patient worse. He only suggested further intervention if there was no

improvement. Because many conditions are self-limiting, the method often worked. A healthy diet and little intervention take up enough time for the condition to get better on its own. The physician is then given credit for the successful outcome.

Nothing will come of nothing?

Most physicians probably knew that the medicines they had to offer would have little genuine effect on the ailments they hoped to cure. They also knew that to retain their credibility (and often their fee) they had to be seen to do something. Although many of the medicines prescribed by early physicians had no physical effect whatsoever, there are numerous accounts of grateful patients claiming that they had been cured. The extensive collection of votary messages and offerings left at the temple of Asclepius demonstrates the power of belief. Hundreds, or even thousands, of people believed that temple sleep and the medicines prescribed by the gods had made them better.

The placebo effect – when an illness is apparently cured because of the patient's belief that they will be cured – is well known to modern medics. Some people see it as a way of explaining the apparent success of conjure and voodoo, prayer, faith healing and perhaps also homeopathy. There have been relatively few studies of the placebo effect, but those that have been conducted show that patients taking sugar pills with no medicinal content often experience an improvement in their condition. In the case of a depressive illness, the success rate for placebos is often little worse than the

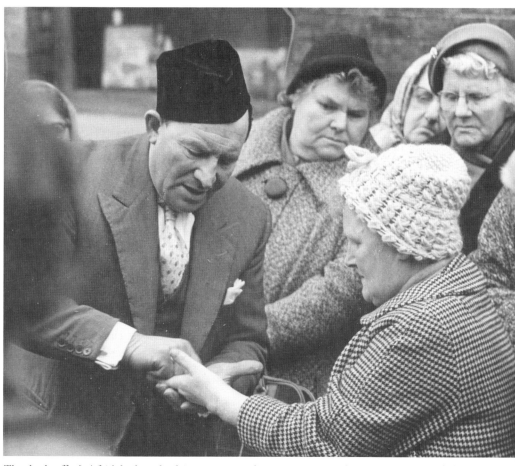

The placebo effect? A faith healer, who claims to summon divine or supernatural intervention on behalf of the ill, draws a crowd of interested ladies in Cheshire, 1963

success rate achieved by antidepressant drugs. Interestingly, the effectiveness of a genuine drug apparently reduces if more successful drugs are discovered (presumably confidence in the original drug decreases) or if the physician has no confidence in the drug (they subconsciously communicate their pessimism to the patient). Injections with no medicinal content (such as salt water) are more effective for reducing pain than sugar pills – simply because an injection is a more invasive and dramatic treatment and patients expect a more dramatic result from it.

Curing like with like

Homeopathy is based on an ancient belief that 'like cures like'. Modern homeopathy developed from the ideas of the German doctor Samuel Hahnemann (1755–1843). He began experimenting with homeopathy in 1790 when he became disillusioned

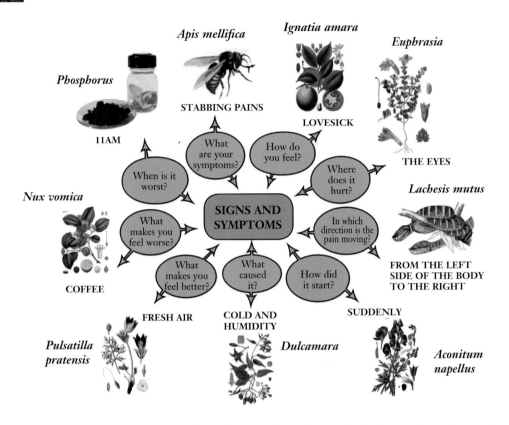

Phosphorus

Apis mellifica

STABBING PAINS

Ignatia amara

LOVESICK

Euphrasia

THE EYES

11AM

Nux vomica

COFFEE

What are your symptoms?

When is it worst?

What makes you feel worse?

How do you feel?

Where does it hurt?

SIGNS AND SYMPTOMS

In which direction is the pain moving?

Lachesis mutus

FROM THE LEFT SIDE OF THE BODY TO THE RIGHT

What makes you feel better?

What caused it?

How did it start?

FRESH AIR

Pulsatilla pratensis

COLD AND HUMIDITY

Dulcamara

SUDDENLY

Aconitum napellus

A sample homeopathic diagnosis tool, showing the active factors to be considered in determining an illness, and which 'mother tincture' should be used in accordance with these factors

with the traditional treatments of bloodletting, purging and the use of toxins such as mercury. He soon became interested in cinchona bark, which is used as a cure for malaria, and he noticed that ingesting the bark caused a malaria-like fever. From this discovery he developed the principle of looking for a substance that exactly produced the symptoms of the disease he wanted to cure.

According to the advocates of homeopathy, the basic substance (or mother tincture) then needs to be diluted. The more dilute the homeopathic preparation is, the more potent it is supposed to be as a medicine. Some homeopathic remedies have been diluted to such

Samuel Hahnemann founded modern-day homeopathy

126

an extent that not a single molecule of the original active ingredient is likely to exist in any one dose. But never mind: water has a 'memory', according to the homeopaths, so it carries the benefit of the substance that was once dissolved in it.

Homeopathy, like many eastern medicines, aims to treat the whole person, not just the disease, so the homeopath takes a full history of the patient. The aim, as in so many much older systems, is to restore the balance of the individual's vital force or energy.

Homeopathy gained popularity and credibility during the 19th century. The homeopathic hospital in London achieved better survival rates than the regular hospitals during the cholera epidemic of 1854, but that did not necessarily mean that the homeopathic remedies were effective. It was perhaps more to do with the fact that the 'remedies' (such as bloodletting) applied by the traditional hospitals were positively harmful.

Much later, in 2007, a great deal of criticism followed claims by homeopaths that they could effectively treat HIV/AIDS and prevent malaria, leading patients to be dangerously negligent of their health. Within days of the outbreak of H1N1 flu from Mexico in 2009, homeopathic treatments and preventives were advertised online. Despite its continuing and growing presence around the world, there is no clinical evidence to support the claims of homeopathy to be effective in these (or indeed any other) areas.

More harm than good?

For thousands of years well-meaning doctors have poisoned and injured their patients, in the name of offering a cure. We might wonder why patients endured this sort of treatment – but perhaps some modern therapies will seem little better to future generations. Many modern patients accept cancer treatments that cause nausea, weakness and hair loss, or take drugs with debilitating side effects, in the hope of a cure. We subject our teenagers to painful orthodontic treatment yet sneer at foot-binding. Every culture has a price that it is willing to pay for the promise of improved health and perceived beauty.

But in some areas the price of relying so heavily on modern drugs has already become too great. The over-use of antibiotics has led to the emergence of resistant strains of disease, for instance. The ease with which doctors have been prescribing antibiotics, along with the routine, prophylactic use of antibiotics in agriculture, has now been called into question. At the end of the first decade of the 21st century doctors are beginning to prescribe fewer of these drugs while suggesting other, non-interventionist therapies. In some cases they are letting minor infections run their course. Hippocrates would be well satisfied.

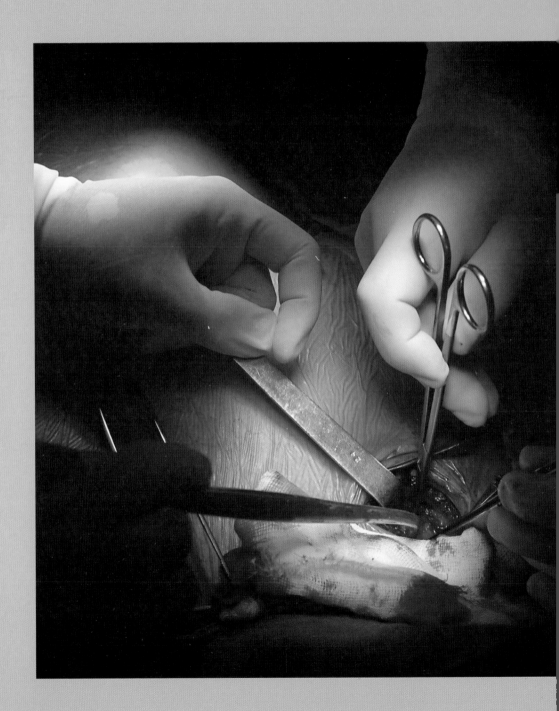

CHAPTER 5

UNDER THE KNIFE

What drugs will not cure, the knife will; what the knife will not cure, the cautery will; what the cautery will not cure must be considered incurable.

Hippocratic Corpus

Throughout most of history, surgery was a terrifying, agonizing and often deadly measure of last resort. With no anaesthesia and no understanding of how infection occurred, only the most desperate patients dared contemplate it – and only the strongest and bravest of surgeons would attempt it. Much surgery was practised *in extremis*: on the battlefield or at sea, where conditions were desperately bad and speed was of the essence (even more so than usual).

It was not until the 19th century, and the development of anaesthesia and antisepsis, that surgery became both endurable and survivable. Surgeons could work at a slower pace and so were able to develop the skills needed for sophisticated procedures. In the 21st century, surgeons no longer just remove the offending part as quickly as possible – they can now often repair or replace diseased or damaged parts. Patients are restored to health rather than just being patched up.

Modern surgery is relatively safe and often highly effective – but it has taken a long time to reach this stage

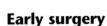

Early surgery

Our primitive ancestors lived dangerous lives, and no doubt injury was common. Falls, fights and attacks by wild animals would produce broken bones, gashes and even lost limbs. It is likely that from the earliest times people learned to bind up cuts, staunch the flow of blood and set bones in some simple manner. Around 8–9,000 years ago humans began to take on more ambitious surgical projects.

DRILLING FOR DEMONS

Skulls with holes in them provide the earliest evidence of invasive surgery. They are the result of an operation known as trepanning or trephining. It is impossible to know exactly how our ancestors hoped this procedure, which sounds more like torture than treatment, would help them. Perhaps they hoped to relieve headaches or pressure in the head by allowing something to escape, such as demons or evil spirits. The 'surgeon' used a flint boring device to make a hole in the skull. Many of the skulls, some dating from 6500BC, show evidence of healing and some have more than one hole – showing that the patient not only survived but also endured the operation for a second, or even a third, time. Trephined skulls have been found in Europe and South America and trephining was still current in parts of Algeria and Melanesia in the 20th century.

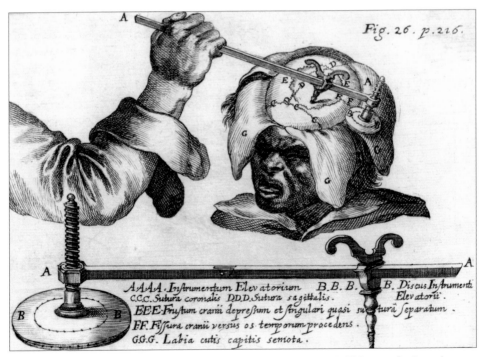

A detailed diagram of an unsavoury-looking trephining operation, circa 1670. Today, a refined – and no doubt less agonizing – model of trephining known as a craniotomy is used to treat brain injuries

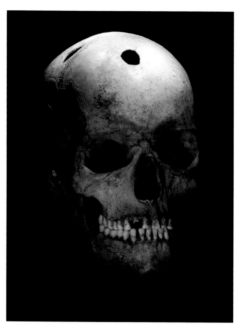

Trephined skulls up to 8,500 years old provide evidence of early surgery

Tools of the trade

The earliest surgical instruments were made of bone, flint, animal horn, sharp shards of shell and shark teeth. Sharp flints were probably used for trephining in prehistoric Europe. In pre-Columbian South America the medical kit contained obsidian knives and spatulas made of sperm whale teeth, while on the Pacific island of Tuvalu shark teeth were used in surgery as recently as 100 years ago. The teeth were inserted into a wooden handle and secured with vegetable fibre in order to make a tool that could be used for bloodletting and scarification, or lancing abscesses. Splinters of bone and antler were probably used as probes by our prehistoric ancestors, and the Cherokee used turkey bone splinters set in a frame of

A HOLE IN THE HEAD
An Englishwoman flew to the United States in 2000, in order to carry out trephining on herself. (The procedure is illegal in the UK but not in the United States.) The woman had suffered from chronic fatigue syndrome for years. Using a local anaesthetic, she stood in front of a mirror and drilled a hole in her head. She needed emergency surgery after drilling too far and perforating a membrane, but she claimed some degree of success. Amateur trephining is not uncommon: many practitioners believe that trephining gives their brain more space and an increased supply of oxygen. Joey Mellen described successfully trephining himself in 1970 in the book *Bore Hole*:

After some time there was an ominous sounding schlurp and the sound of bubbling. I drew the trepan out and the gurgling continued. It sounded like air bubbles running under the skull as they were pressed out. I looked at the trepan and there was a bit of bone in it. At last!

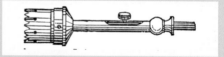

A tool used for removing a portion of the skull during a trephining operation

turkey quills as a scarificator. Hollow bones have been used as canulas in several societies. The Fijians used the metacarpal bone of a flying fox to produce a tube that was used to drain fluid from the scrotum. In Blanche Bay, New Britain, the wing bones of a flying fox were sharpened and used in trephining operations.

Once people learned to work with metal they used it to make surgical instruments. Copper surgical instruments were used in ancient Egypt. The Arabs made particularly fine metal tools more than 1,000 years ago, the designs of which have been refined over the ensuing centuries (see p.136). Many new designs have emerged in response to advances in surgical techniques; instruments are now made almost exclusively from stainless steel. Since the advent of microsurgery, surgeons have begun to use tiny robotically controlled tools, manipulated with the aid of an operating microscope.

Some tools can no longer be laid on an instrument tray, but disappear when the electricity supply is turned off. Laser tweezers and scalpels are beams of intense energy which are powerful enough to pick up or nudge cells, or cut through tissue. Ultrasound – high energy sound – is a painless way in which to blast apart the bladder stones that caused such agony to early lithotomy patients, as well as the gallstones and the kidney stones that early surgeons could not treat at all. Radiation is used to destroy cancerous cells, and, prompted by curious MRI side effects, recent studies undertaken now suggest that magnetism may be useful in treating depression.

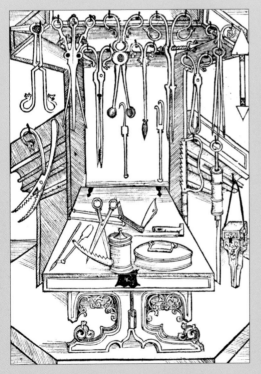

TOOLS FOR THE SURGEON'S CHEST

In 1617 ship's surgeon John Woodall created a chilling list of tools and instruments to be included in every surgeon's chest. It comprised 'Incision knives, Dismembring knives, Catlings, Rasours [razors], Trapans [drills for trephining], Head Sawes, Dismembring Sawes, Dismembring Nippers, Mallet and Chizell, and Cauterizing irons'. He comments:

It is commendable in an Artist [surgeon] to be very carefull to hide his sharpe instruments (as much as is possible) from the sight of the Patient, for many reasons too long to recite.

A grim array of tools in the surgeon's chest awaits the unlucky patient

THE EDWIN SMITH PAPYRUS – CASE 33, BROKEN NECK
Instructions concerning a crushed vertebra in his neck.

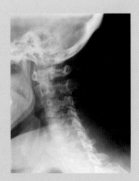

If thou examinest a man having a crushed vertebra in his neck [and] thou findest that one vertebra has fallen into the next one, while he is voiceless and cannot speak; his falling head downward has caused that one vertebra to crush into the next one; [and] shouldst thou find that he is unconscious of his two arms and his two legs because of it...

Thou shouldst say concerning him: 'One having a crushed vertebra in his neck; he is unconscious of his two arms [and] his two legs, [and] he is speechless. An ailment not to be treated.'...

A broken or dislocated neck is hard to treat, even today

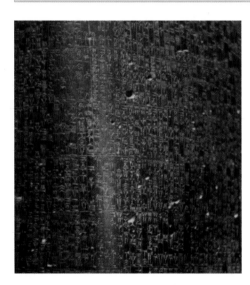

The laws of Hammurabi are preserved on a stone stela in the Louvre, Paris

Doctors vs. surgeons

For at least 4,000 years there was a distinction between doctors who dealt in medicine (and often spells) and surgeons who carried out procedures. Doctor-priests usually had a higher status than surgeons, who were often seen as little more than skilled mechanics of the body, working with their hands rather than their brains. Assyrian and Babylonian doctors were answerable to the gods, but surgeons were laymen governed by ordinary law. The Code of Hammurabi, the earliest surviving legal code, recorded some of the rules that covered the activities of surgeons (see p.174).

Mummies and medics

The Edwin Smith Papyrus (c.1600BC) deals with 48 cases, mostly of trauma, and divides them into three categories, in a way that is similar to modern triage: 'an ailment which I will treat', 'an ailment with which I will contend', and 'an ailment not to be treated'.

Other early texts also include references to surgical procedures.

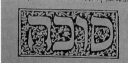

The Talmud, an ancient Hebrew text

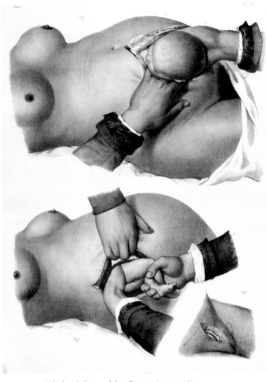

A baby delivered by Caesarian section

The Hebrew Talmud (The Mishnah, 70–200) contains descriptions of operations for anal fistula and Caesarean section, and explains how to set fractures. It even describes an incident of cranial surgery. The account tells how a man with a now-unidentifiable disease called *ra'atan* has his skull opened and some 'organism' scraped from the *meninges* (the membrane covering the brain). Before the operation, 300 cups of a herbal brew were poured over the head, perhaps as some kind of anaesthetic. The operation was carried out in a marble room with no draught, which suggests an awareness of infection coming from unclean conditions. The text specifies that all of the 'organism' must be removed or the condition will return.

Indian surgery

The *Susruta Samhita* describes an extensive range of surgical procedures and lists 121 surgical instruments in use around 600BC, including knives, scissors, tweezers, catheters, needles and magnets for removing metal objects. Susruta describes operations to treat anal fistulas and tumours in the neck. He explains how to remove the tonsils and the prostate gland; amputate limbs; lance abscesses; use bamboo splints to set broken bones; suture wounds (including intestinal wounds); remove teeth; and take foreign bodies from the nose and the ear.

One of Susruta's most famous procedures was the reconstruction of noses, earlobes and cleft lips – the first known instance of reconstructive or plastic surgery. In Susruta's India, adultery was punished by cutting off the offender's nose, so surgeons had a good supply of patients. Susruta explained how to rebuild a nose using grafted skin from the forehead or the cheek, only cutting the flap free when the graft had taken. He used wine to intoxicate his patients, which dulled the pain and made them compliant. It seems that not just surgeons but also tilemakers and potters of the Koomas caste undertook the operation. In their case they took the skin from the buttock, first beating it with a paddle until it was red. Clearly in this case the skin could not be left attached while the graft took.

The Italian Gaspare Tagliacozzi (1546–99), used a similar procedure. A flap of skin on the patient's arm was lifted   and

HOW TO BUILD A NOSE

Susruta's instructions for rhinoplasty tell the surgeon to begin by laying a leaf on the cheek of the patient. The surgeon should cut around the leaf, lift the skin and then stitch the skin flap over the nose stump. He should then insert two reeds to allow the patient to breathe by acting as nostrils. They would also give the nose some shape. If, after this, the nose was too large, he should cut it off and start again.

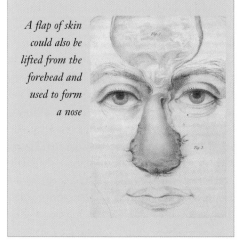

A flap of skin could also be lifted from the forehead and used to form a nose

the arm was then strapped to the head until the graft was secure – after that, the flap was cut free. Tagliacozzi was the first doctor to make the technique well known in Europe. Two families in Calabria and one in Sicily practised rhinoplasty from around 1400, but they guarded the procedure as a family secret. Tagliacozzi might have done better to have followed their example: he was charged with impious behaviour and the operation was banned, not to be allowed again until 1822.

Classical surgeons

The Hippocratic writings say surgery is to be avoided if possible – it should only be used as a final resort. Even then the doctor should eschew it – most operations should be left to professional surgeons. Some simple and essential procedures are described, including setting broken bones and lancing boils. There is some discussion of cutting out nasal polyps and ulcerated tonsils, but the removal of bladder stones (lithotomy) was always carried out by surgical craftsmen who specialized in this single operation.

Greek culture continued to flourish in Hellenic Alexandria after its decline in Greece. Many Hellenic doctors went from Alexandria to Rome. The Romans initially disdained practical medicine, preferring to depend on magic, superstition and religion. They railed against the Greek doctors who flocked to Rome in large numbers in the 3rd and 2nd centuries BC. Pliny records that Cato (234–149BC) considered Greek doctors a threat to Roman health and claimed that they intended to kill Romans. As Cato promoted cabbages as the cure for all ills that were not amenable to prayer and magic, it is hard to see how the Greeks could present much more of a threat than he did himself. Even so, the Romans came around to the idea eventually and Julius Caesar granted Roman citizenship to foreign doctors. Surgery was practised in Rome, despite the reservations of Cato: Asclepiades of Prusa is credited with performing a tracheotomy in the 1st century BC (perhaps in a case of diptheria) and Celsus gave the first account of lithotomy in the 1st century AD.

When Paul of Aegina compiled *Epitomae medicae libri septem (Medical Compendium in Seven Books)* he brought together the legacy of the great classical Greek physicians and surgeons and added some of his own unique developments. His text included a volume on surgery, which covers the techniques for tracheotomy, tonsillectomy, catheterizing the bladder, removing bladder stones, repairing inguinal hernias and breast reduction. The *Epitomae* probably dates from around the 7th century AD; it influenced great Arab doctors such as Rhazes, Abulcasis, Haly Abbas and Avicenna.

Surgery in the Arab world

There were 800 doctors in 9th-century Baghdad. Between them, they pioneered new surgical techniques and developed new tools. The skill of Arab metalworkers enabled the production of fine and beautifully elegant tools which made delicate operations such as lifting and suturing blood vessels possible for the first time. Many of the Arab designs of surgical instruments are still in use, having changed little in over 1,000 years. They were first described in the 10th century by the so-called 'father of surgery' Abu al-Qasim al-Zahrawi (Abulcasis) (c.936–1013). In his encyclopedic medical texts he described his collection of more than 200 surgical instruments. Twenty-six of them had never been described before so they might have been his own invention, including forceps, speculum, curette, scalpel, surgical needle, hook and spoon. He also introduced the use of cat gut for internal stitches, as the only material that would dissolve naturally in the body.

The fourth book of Avicenna's five-volume *Canon*, written in the 11th century, included a treatise on surgery. When it was translated into Latin in the 13th century by Gerard of Cremona or Gerard de Sabloneta, it became the second most authoritative medical text after Galen's works. But the Arabs made greater advances in pharmacology and other aspects of medicine than in surgery, which they generally held in low regard. When

---

ASCLEPIADES OF PRUSA (2ND/1ST CENTURY BC)

Asclepiades was born in Bythnia and died in Rome. He practised medicine in several places in between, including Parium and Athens. Pliny reports that he made a wager with fortune that he should not be considered a proper physician if he ever fell ill himself: he won the wager, finally dying in old age by falling downstairs. He was said to have founded a new medical school and to have discovered a way of preparing wine for patients which was very popular with them. He also developed a type of swinging bed, which was used to lull patients to sleep. According to Pliny, Asclepiades advocated only five treatments: fasting, abstention from wine, massage, walking and carriage rides (!). On one occasion he is said to have stopped a passing funeral procession and revived the supposedly dead man being carried to burial.

TREATMENT OF VARICOSE VEINS – PAUL OF AEGINA

[H]aving washed the man, and applied a ligature round the upper part of the thigh, we are to direct him to walk about, and when the vein becomes distended we are to mark its situation with writing ink, to the extent of three fingers' breadth or a little more, and having placed the man in a reclining posture with his leg extended, we apply another ligature above the knee; and where the vein is distended we make an incision upon the mark with a scalpel, but not to a greater depth than the thickness of the skin, lest we divide the vein; and having separated the lips of the wound with hooks, and dissected away the membranes with crooked specilla, like those used in the operation of hydrocele, and laid bare the vein, and freed it all around, we loose the ligatures from the thigh, and having raised the vessel with a blind hook, and introduced under it a needle having a double thread we cut the double of it, and opening the vein in the middle with a lancet, evacuate as much blood as may be required. Then having tied the upper part of the vessel with one of the ligatures, and stretched the leg, we evacuate the blood in the limb by compression with the hands. Then having tied the lower part of the vein, we may either cut out the portion intermediate between the ligatures, or suffer it to remain until it drop out of its own accord with the ligatures; then we have to put a dry pledget into the wound, and apply over it an oblong compress soaked in wine and oil, and secure them with a bandage... I am aware that some of the ancients do not use ligatures, but cut out the vessel immediately after it is laid bare, whilst others stretch it from below and tear it out by force. But the mode of operating now described is of all others the safest.

Epitomae, Book 6

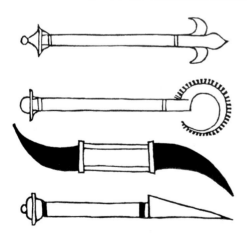

Arab medical instruments from the encyclopedia
Al-Tasrif (The Method of Medicine), *written*
around AD1000

Abulcasis asked himself why the Arabs had not made more progress in the field of surgery, he decided that a lack of anatomical knowledge and an insufficient study of Galen had held them back.

Monks, surgeons and barber-surgeons

In Europe, from around AD500, monks had performed simple techniques such as blood-letting, lancing abscesses and extracting teeth, but in 1163 a papal edict prohibited them from practising any type of surgery. Barbers often assisted the monks in their procedures; they came to the monasteries to shave the monks, and their sharp tools came

ABU AL-QASIM AL-ZAHRAWI (ABULCASIS) (c.936–1013)

The greatest medieval Arab surgeon, Abulcasis, was born in El Zahra in Moorish Spain. Reputed as the 'father of surgery', he spent most of his life in nearby Córdoba, where his house is still preserved (number 6, Calle Albucasis). According to an account of his life written 60 years

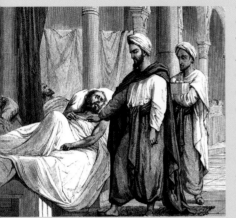

after his death, he practised and taught medicine in Córdoba during the whole of his working life, and also worked as court physician to the Andalusian caliph Al-Hakan II. He is most famous for his 30-volume encyclopedia, *Kitab al-Tasrif*, which covers all aspects of surgery, medicine, pharmacology, obstetrics, ophthalmology, dentistry and nutrition and is the first illustrated medical text. His work was translated into Latin by Gerard of Cremona in the 12th century and it was used throughout Europe and the Middle East for at least 500 years. Abulcasis was the first doctor to describe an ectopic pregnancy, in which the foetus develops outside the uterus, usually in a fallopian tube. He was also the first to refer to the hereditary nature of haemophilia.

Abulcasis attending a patient in the hospital at Córdoba

in useful. When the monks were no longer allowed to carry out surgical procedures, the barbers took over the role, becoming barber-surgeons. In 1210, the first guild of barbers was formed in France to regulate the profession. Barber-surgeons continued to carry out everyday procedures until the 18th century.

From the 11th century onwards, the surgical knowledge amassed by the Greeks and the Arabs spread slowly through Europe, starting in Spain and Italy. The division between surgeons and barber-surgeons was clearest in their relationship to this learning. The barber-surgeons trained in a physical skill through apprenticeship and practice and they dealt with simple, everyday procedures such as blood-letting, setting broken limbs, binding up wounds and lancing boils. 'True' surgeons, whose numbers were gradually increasing, studied at one of the medical schools. The first school was founded at Salerno in Italy and others followed in Italy and France. These specialist doctors had a theoretical knowledge of how the body was thought to work, they learned Latin and

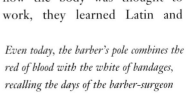

Even today, the barber's pole combines the red of blood with the white of bandages, recalling the days of the barber-surgeon

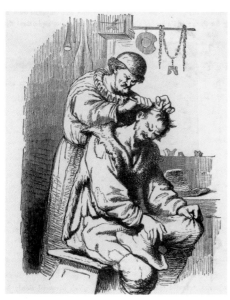

A 17th-century barber-surgeon performing an
operation on a patient

Greek and they increasingly had a knowledge of anatomy that was drawn from dissection. European surgeons published new works, although they still drew heavily on the ancient authorities. One of the most influential medical texts of the Middle Ages was the encyclopedic *Chirurgia magna* of Guy de Chauliac, which included treatment for cataract and hernia. It remained the principal authority on surgical procedures from its composition in 1363 until the 17th century.

A series of laws passed in the 15th century limited the procedures that barber-surgeons could undertake, crystallizing the distinction between the two kinds of medical practitioners and contributing to the rise in prestige of the learned surgeons. At the same time, groups of itinerant specialists travelled from place to place carrying out a single procedure, such as lithotomy (removing bladder stones), cataract removal or hernia repairs. These itinerant practitioners continued to make a living amongst poorer and rural patients, while from the 16th century onwards professional, trained surgeons began to take a hold in the cities.

Although a few medieval surgeons like de Chauliac pioneered new techniques, the great advances in surgery were made after the Renaissance. Increasingly, the more menial aspects of surgery fell into the laps of the barber-surgeons, leaving the trained surgeons to higher pursuits, including anatomical research. But until the watershed of the mid 19th century, when anaesthetics and antisepsis revolutionized surgery of all types, the day-to-day practice of surgery was limited to dealing with traumatic injury and treating a limited range of fairly straightforward (if often fatal) problems. Abdominal surgery was very rarely attempted and was almost always lethal.

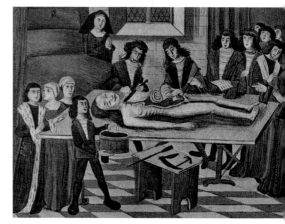

Guy de Chauliac demonstrating the surgical
procedures that he pioneered

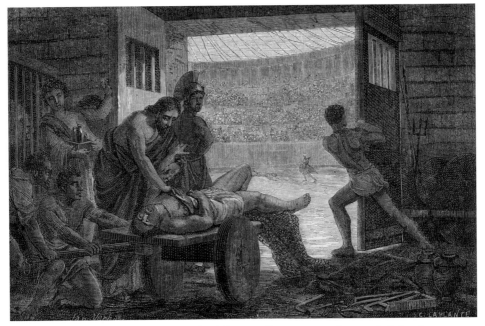

Galen learnt his trade as chief physician to the gladiators at Pergamum – so he never lacked patients on whom to practise his skills

Surgeons and soldiers

From the time of Hippocrates, and probably before, surgery had been closely linked with soldiering and war. Battles produced wounds of many types which demanded a rapid medical response, often in terrible conditions. Surgeons who had trained on the battlefield, and later on ships, were the best, as Herodotus noted: 'He who wishes to be a surgeon should go to war.' The Roman physician Galen was a surgeon to gladiators, and Paul of Aegina wrote extensively about treating injuries from war weapons. Later, Paracelsus worked with the Dutch and Venetian armies as a surgeon, and Vesalius and Paré worked on opposite sides of the walls during the siege of Saint-Dizier, when France and the forces of the Holy Roman Emperor were at war in 1544.

The experience gained from treating injuries sustained in wartime gave surgeons the expertise to treat similar wounds sustained in everyday life.

Injuries from early weapons such as swords, spears, arrows and slingshots provided plenty of opportunities for the surgeon to develop his skills. Wounds could include sword slashes; severed limbs; sharp objects that had pierced, or become embedded in, the body; fractures; crushed bones; dislocated joints; lacerations; and burns – all part of the daily fare of a surgeon to the army or the navy. With the arrival of gunpowder from the Far East in the later Middle Ages, war wounds took on a new, horrific dimension. Injuries from gunshot and cannon were gruesome, and lead bullets carried foreign material far into the body,

---

MEND AND MAKE DO – TREATING WOUNDS

Surgeons had to operate quickly to remove foreign bodies, splint and bind wounds, relocate joints, staunch bleeding and amputate smashed or infected limbs. Even with speedy treatment, filthy conditions often led to infection. Hippocrates taught that a wound suppurating with pus was a healthy wound (he called it 'laudable pus'), and this advice doubtless led to many deaths. It was not until the Middle Ages that surgeons began to challenge received wisdom. Among them were Guy de Chauliac and Henri de Mondeville (b.1260), who both recommended the dry treatment of wounds, instead of encouraging the formation of pus.

---

frequently causing infection. Indeed, infection was so common that for many years surgeons believed that a wound caused by firearms was actually poisoned by the weapon itself.

The ancient Egyptians recognized that a wound must be kept free from infection. Even though they did not understand the processes they were employing, they managed to exclude bacteria and provide a framework for reconstruction. The Ebers Papyrus (c.1500BC) tells how wounds were treated with animal grease and honey before covering them with lint. The grease provided a barrier against the air and kept in moisture, the honey had antibiotic properties, and the lint provided a fibrous base for closure. The Greeks and the Romans also used honey on wounds, and it was still in use during both world wars. Recent research suggests that honey is effective in treating wounds infected by antibiotic-resistant bacteria. The antibacterial effect is produced by an enzyme that makes hydrogen peroxide (an antiseptic) from sugar.

A wound crawling with maggots may look disgusting but it's actually pretty healthy. Australian Aborigines, the Burmese hill people and the Mayans all deliberately

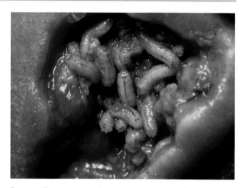

Larva therapy in action: an open wound being cleaned by surgical maggots

---

RUBBING SALT IN THE WOUND

The ancient Egyptians, Greeks and Romans all used salt on wounds. It was intended to dry them out and it helped to prevent infection. The ancient Egyptians also urinated on wounds (urine contains salt, and it is sterile). Although salt stings on open wounds, it does encourage clean healing. During the Second World War, the New Zealand doctor Sir Archibald McIndoe introduced the use of a saline bath to treat burns. He had noticed that the burns of pilots who were shot down over the sea healed better than those of pilots who had been shot down over land.

EATEN ALIVE!

In modern larva therapy, greenbottle larvae bred in sterile conditions eat away pus and rotting flesh and provide antibiotics at the same time. Enzymes in the maggots' saliva dissolve the organic tissue and kill bacteria, and the maggots suck up the resultant gooey soup. They crawl into all the nooks and crannies of a wound to clean it efficiently. Maggots also seem to produce a secretion that kick-starts healing; scientists at the University of Nottingham are investigating this aspect. In some cases, maggots have apparently eaten away cancerous tumours.

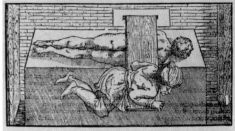

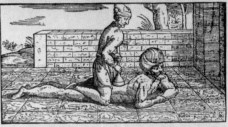

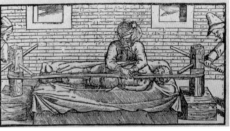

Early treatment for a spinal dislocation included exerting pressure using leverage (top), pounding with a heavy instrument (middle) and traction (bottom)

introduced maggots into wounds to help clean them. Napoleon's battlefield surgeon Baron Dominique-Jean Larrey noticed in the 1820s that injured soldiers did well if their wounds became infested with maggots. During the First World War, surgeon William S. Baer discovered that two men who had lain on the battlefield for a week and had maggot-infested wounds were free from infection and gangrene. Following his research in the late 1920s, maggots were used in over 300 hospitals in North America. The arrival of antibiotics drove out maggots, but in the wake of antibiotic-resistant infections maggots are again attracting attention and fans under the sanitized name of 'larva therapy'.

Baron Dominique-Jean Larrey was an important innovator in battlefield medicine

All at sea

Going to sea was a dangerous occupation. Apart from the usual illnesses and accidents that might befall anyone, sailors suffered from an appalling diet and were prone to injuries while working the ship or when they were in battle. The ship's surgeon was a vital member of the community

TREATING THE SWORD

In the 17th century, Sir Kenelm Digby made popular a 'wound salve' for treating sword wounds. It was concocted from a fabulous mix of ingredients including ground earthworms, pig's brains, Egyptian mummy and iron oxide. The salve was to be applied to the sword that had made the wound rather than to the wound itself. Its popularity doubtless owes something to the fact that it caused no additional pain to the patient and it was probably no less efficient than many other treatments. However, locating the offending sword must often have proved difficult.

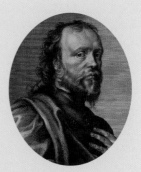

Sir Kenelm Digby

who was overworked in times of battle and stretched the rest of the time. In 1617 John Woodall, a surgeon at St Bartholomew's Hospital in London, published the first edition of his extensive handbook for physicians practising on board ship. He recommended washing tools and dressings in vinegar, a primitive method of sterilizing them, and using 'restrictive' powder to staunch bleeding. Blood from operations should be caught in a bowl filled with ashes, which would soak it up – a wise precaution on a rocking ship where a bowl might easily overturn. The dismembering saw, he said, must be kept wrapped in oiled cloth to prevent it rusting. Much of the surgeon's work involved removing shot and debris from injured sailors. If a wound went gangrenous, as it often did, the limb must be amputated. Instead of the usual brutal sawing and cutting through the living flesh above the gangrene, Woodall advised a new and less aggressive method of amputation. He recommended first cutting through the dead, gangrenous flesh, which does not hurt the patient. Then the surgeon should test for feeling with a needle and cut and

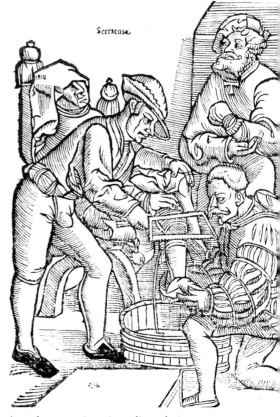

An early amputation using a dismembering saw, with the surgeon in his ordinary clothes. Unsurprisingly, the patient mortality rate was high

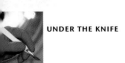

AN AMPUTATION

The patient is first prepared so that he can give informed consent to the procedure:

> *If you be constrained to use your Saw, let first your Patient be well informed of the eminent danger of death the use thereof; prescribe him no certaintie of life, and let the work be done with his owne free will, and request; and not otherwise. Let him prepare his soule as a ready sacrifice to the Lord by earnest prayers, craving mercie and helpe from the Almightie, and that heartily. For it is no small presumption to Dismember the Image of God.*

Then the surgeon turns to the terrible deed:

> *Take your dismembering knife, and with a steddy hand and good speed, cut off flesh, sinewes and all, to the bone round about the member, which done, take a smaller incision knife and divide the panicle called the* periosteon, *from the bone, it is a tough thin skin, covering all the bones of the body; also thrust your said incision knife betwixt the fossels or bones, cutting away whatsoever is to bee found there with like expedition: the partie [man] that holdeth the upper part of the legge with all his strength, griping the member together to keepe in the spirits and bloud: It were also very good that the said party holding the member, the flesh and sinewes being cut asunder, should immediately draw or strip upward the flesh so much as he could, keeping his hold, that thereby the Saw may come so much the neerer, which would occasion a quicker and better healing, the flesh being thereby made longer then the end of the bone: then if you approve of that course of stitching, as some good men do, take the two strong square needle & threds mentioned, and presently after the member is taken away, stitch the skin thorow on the one side, and just over on the other side, and with the other needle doe likewise as it were crosse over the member the other way, & draw the said threds so close as you think convenient, the better to stop and choake the great veines & arteries.*

John Woodall, *The Surgeon's Mate*, 1639

burn away the dead flesh an inch from the point where the flesh is live.

This, usefully, required only three assistants, whereas amputation through live flesh needed five assistants to attend the surgeon and restrain the patient. Later, any extra dead flesh should be removed using cauterizing irons and scissors. Woodall was adamant that a surgeon must be as conservative as possible in amputation:

> *... for the offence or disease of the toes, let onley the toes suffer, and no more of the members of the body be lost... it is just that so much be amputated as deserveth expulsion, and not, as is said, to take away a sound and blameless legge, when it is innocent and free from fault, errour, or disease.*

The business of surgery

Even in peacetime, surgery was a final option. Shunned and feared, it was something to be resorted to when death had become the only alternative. Despite this, plenty of accounts have survived. Some of them are instructions for practitioners and others are patient or witness testimonies to the horrors of undergoing surgery. Most procedures were quick and relatively simple – but that did not make them any less of an ordeal.

CATARACT SURGERY

A technique called couching has long been used to remove cataracts. It involves inserting a needle through the white of the eye and dislodging, or sometimes breaking up, the clouded lens that obscures vision. The lens (or part of it) falls to the bottom of the eye, allowing light to penetrate again. Although the lens allows the eye to vary its focus, it is not essential to vision. Couching was first described by Celsus in AD29. One Roman writer reported that it had been developed when a blind goat had been seen to have its sight restored after running into a thorn. The Indian surgeon Susruta described making an incision in the eye and pushing the cataract

downwards, out of the way. Arab surgeons practised couching extensively, even until the middle of the 20th century in some areas. In around AD1000, Ammar ibn Ali al-Mawsili described using a hollow needle supposedly to suck the cataract from the eye, although others failed to make this technique work. This is the first reference to a hypodermic needle.

Eventually, couching was replaced by an operation to make an incision in the eye and remove the lens (initially without anaesthetic) by scooping it out with a spatula. This operation was first performed by Jacques Daviel in Paris, France, in 1747. It was not always successful: the composer Handel was one of the patients who was left blind when the procedure went wrong. Later refinements included using pressure to squeeze out the lens and a suction cup to suck it out. The invention of cocaine eye drops as an anaesthetic in 1884 made the process less traumatic for the patient and easier for the surgeon. Nearly a hundred years went by before the next major breakthrough. In 1967 Charles Kelman (1930–2004) banished the scalpel completely. He used ultrasound to blast the cataract to bits and then the debris was sucked from the eye. Modern cataract

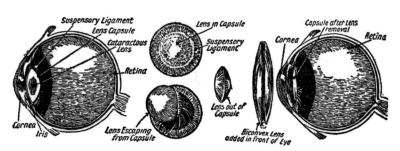

Diagrams showing the removal of the lens during early cataract surgery – performed without anaesthetic

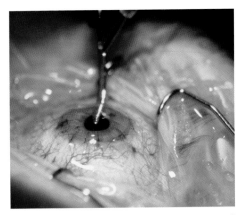

Modern cataract surgery is made easier by the use of anaesthetics. It also allows for insertion of an acrylic lens to improve the patient's quality of vision

surgery replaces the damaged lens with an artificial acrylic lens, which provides sharper vision than the earlier techniques could offer.

CUTTING FOR THE STONE

Bladder stones cause excruciating pain, but so did the operation to remove them – 'cutting for the stone' (lithotomy). The procedure is first recorded in Greece at the time of Hippocrates (c.460–c.375 BC), though doctors did not carry it out themselves but left it to specialists. Aulus Cornelius Celsus gave the first account of the operation in the 1st century AD. He described a method of cutting through the perinium that would be used until the middle of the 16th century, at least for children.

In about 1520 a new method of perineal lithotomy was devised. This involved inserting a rod into the urethra up to the bladder and then gaining access to the bladder by making an incision in the

perineum, cutting against the rod. The stone was extracted through the incision using forceps. If it was too large it was first crushed and then it was scooped out. The operation was dangerous as well as traumatic. The great surgeon Hermann Boerhaave (1668–1738) considered lithotomy 'an act of pure faith'. Most surgeons resorted to it only when the patient appeared to be in imminent danger of death and all attempts at evacuating the stone had failed.

The horror of the operation made a lasting impact on many patients. The English diarist Samuel Pepys endured an operation for the stone in 1658. He kept the stone in a jar as a memento and ever afterwards he observed the date (26th March) as a holiday. The French composer Marin Marais (1656–1728) even wrote a musical depiction of the operation for

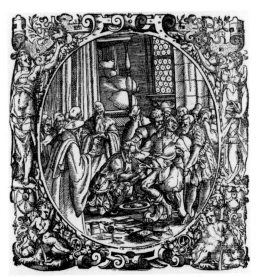

A perineal lithotomy – an operation carried out to remove painful stones from the bladder tract – depicted around 1565

FRÈRE JACQUES (1651–1714)

The itinerant lithotomist known as Frère Jacques travelled around France and Italy between 1690 and 1714. In that time he performed 4,500 lithotomies. Born Jacques Beaulieu, the son of humble Burgundian peasants, he served as a trooper in the cavalry until the age of 21, when he became the servant of a travelling lithotomist. He then learned the trade himself, adopted the robes of a monk (though he was not trained or ordained) and applied for a licence to operate. This was denied, even though he performed a successful lithotomy demonstration on a corpse. However, the king later granted him a royal licence to 'cut for the stone'. His operations were so quick and spectacular that in his heyday he operated before 200 spectators, who bought tickets to watch him 'perform'. He practised successfully until 1698, when he hit a run of bad luck and killed seven patients in one day. After that he learned some badly-needed anatomy and went on to practise more successfully. He refined the technique that was generally used for lithotomy at the time and rebuilt his reputation.

bladder stones in 1725, entitled *Tableau de l'opération de la taille (Picture of a lithotomy)*.

DRAWING TEETH

Only the agony of continuing toothache would induce anyone to have their teeth removed without anaesthetic. The procedure is so painful that it has been used as a form of torture for millennia. On account of the poor dental hygiene of most people throughout history, though, it has often been a necessary evil. In earlier days, teeth were pulled using instruments like pliers, which were

Samuel Pepys survived not only the Great Fire of London, but also a harrowing lithotomy

made by blacksmiths or armourers. These developed into more sophisticated dental forceps, at least for the wealthier practitioner and patient. In the 14th century, Guy de Chauliac introduced the 'dental pelican'. The next development was the 'tooth key', which looked rather like a door key and operated something like a bottle opener. A good deal of twisting was involved in pulling the tooth, and part of the jaw would often break away with it if the tooth was not thoroughly decayed. If a tooth broke during extraction the barber-surgeon would have to dig out the bits separately. Dentists had to be strong and they needed to employ at least one sturdy assistant to hold the patient down.

MAJOR SURGERY

Lithotomy, dentistry and cataract surgery must have been a horrendous ordeal for the patient, but they were relatively straightforward procedures. Major surgery, such as amputations and the excision of tumours, was harrowing for both patient

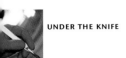

OPEN WIDE

The first reference to dental health is in a Sumerian text from 5000BC, which blames 'tooth worms' for causing decay. An Egyptian tomb dating from 2600BC contains the first known dentist – a scribe called Hesy-Re, who was said to 'deal with teeth'.

Both Hippocrates and Aristotle refer to extracting teeth with forceps, treating decayed teeth and wiring loose teeth to stabilize them. In the 2nd century the Etruscans developed crowns and bridges. Presumably some of the patients who had endured extractions needed bridges, as well as those whose teeth had fallen out.

The first book devoted entirely to dentistry, *Artzney Buchlein*, was published in Germany in 1530. Dentistry had not separated itself as a profession at this stage. In 1575 the French surgeon Ambroise Paré covered the subject in his works, including extraction and treating decay. Dentistry became a separate and respectable profession in 1728, with the publication of Pierre Fouchard's *Le Chirurgien Dentiste*. Fouchard identified sugar as a source of the tartaric acid that causes decay, and he introduced dental fillings.

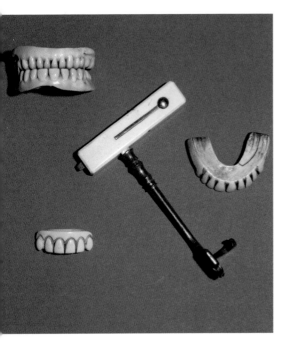

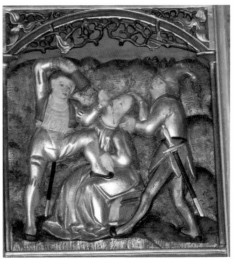

St Apollonia suffering martyrdom, having her teeth drawn (without anaesthetic)

Early dentures and a tooth key, used for extractions. The tooth key, forged from ivory and metal, was used from the 18th century right up to the 20th century, when it was rendered obsolete by the invention of forceps

and practitioner. Tumours could be destroyed by cauterization or they could be cut out. Sometimes the treatment was so successful that the patient survived for many years. It is not possible to overstate the enormity of the undertaking, though.

FALSE TEETH

Bone, jade, precious metals and even wood have all been used to supply false teeth. It is commonly believed that George Washington had wooden dentures, but in fact they were made from gold, lead and ivory, together with human and animal teeth. Donkey and horse teeth, as well as teeth from human corpses, were commonly used in sets of dentures. Washington owned other sets of false teeth, including one made from walrus ivory, which he called his 'sea horse teeth'. The trade in second-hand teeth was such that looters ransacked the battlefields of the Napoleonic wars with pliers, pulling teeth from fallen soldiers.

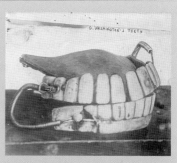

George Washington's false teeth were said to have been soaked in port to suppress the taste of metal, ivory and animal teeth

FANNY BURNEY'S MASTECTOMY

The English novelist and diarist Fanny Burney had a mastectomy without anaesthetic in 1811. It was carried out by Baron de Larrey, surgeon to Napoleon Bonaparte. She described it in a letter written nine months later:

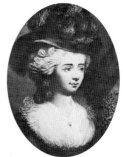

Fanny Burney survived the torture of mastectomy

[I felt] a terror that surpasses all description, & the most torturing pain. Yet – when the dreadful steel was plunged into the breast – cutting through veins – arteries – flesh – nerves – I needed no injunctions not to restrain my cries. I began a scream that lasted unintermittingly during the whole time of the incision – & I almost marvel that it rings not in my Ears still! so excruciating was the agony. When the wound was made, & the instrument was withdrawn, the pain seemed undiminished, for the air that suddenly rushed into those delicate parts felt like a mass of minute but sharp & forked poniards, that were tearing the edges of the wound – but when again I felt the instrument – describing a curve – cutting against the grain, if I may so say, while the flesh resisted in a manner so forcible as to oppose & tire the hand of the operator, who was forced to change from the right to the left – then, indeed, I thought I must have expired... The instrument this second time withdrawn, I concluded the operation over – Oh no! presently the terrible cutting was renewed – & worse than ever, to separate the bottom, the foundation of this dreadful gland from the parts to which it adhered – Again all description would be baffled – yet again all was not over, – Dr Larry rested but his own hand, & – Oh Heaven! – I then felt the Knife tackling against the breast bone – scraping it! – This performed, while I yet remained in utterly speechless torture.

Finishing off

When surgeons – or accidents – make holes in bodies, it is necessary to stop the flow of blood and seal the hole up as quickly as possible. Two methods have been used since early times for staunching bleeding. The ends of the cut vessels must be sealed, either by cauterization or by using a ligature. Then the edges of the wound must be drawn together and held in place until, with luck, the gash heals.

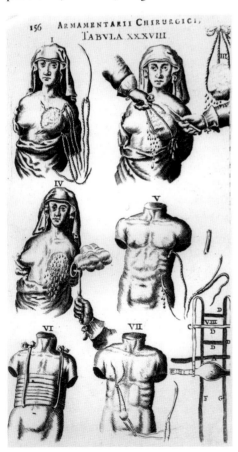

A series of pictures showing how to carry out a radical mastectomy, including the excruciating – and often fatal – process of cauterization

FIRE AND BRIMSTONE

The quickest way to seal a large wound is by cauterizing it, which usually means burning it with a red-hot iron, molten metal or boiling oil. In battle and other emergency situations hot oil was poured into the wound, or a large iron was heated and placed across it. The treatment was so violent that patients already suffering shock from their first traumatic injury often died as a result of the cauterization. In the less frantic atmosphere of planned surgery, doctors used a range of cauters of different sizes. These metal tools were heated in a fire and applied to the wound. Arab surgeons had beautifully crafted cauters. Cauterization was also used to destroy tumours from the time of Hippocrates.

Cauterization was the worst nightmare of soldiers and sailors, worse even than the traumatic injuries that might have necessitated its use. It was finally abandoned in Europe after the great French surgeon Ambroise Paré discovered a kinder method. According to tradition, he made his discovery by accident while working as a novice surgeon with the French army at the siege of Turin in 1536–7. Paré had been told to treat his soldiers with a mixture of hot elder oil and treacle to cauterize their wounds; it would supposedly kill the poison that was thought to be present in wounds caused by gunshot. Paré was reluctant to do it because of the pain it must cause his patients. He went ahead, though, but when he ran out of oil he used instead a soothing mixture of egg yolk, oil of roses and turpentine. Worried that his patients would suffer as a result, he visited them early the next morning to check on their progress.

AMBROISE PARÉ (c.1517–90)

Ambroise Paré's father and uncle were both barber-surgeons, so although he was ill-educated he was well apprenticed. He began his career in Paris, first as a barber-surgeon and then as a house surgeon at the Hôtel-Dieu hospital. After that he became an army surgeon, a role he would carry out for around 30 years. At the siege of Turin, Italy, in 1536 he had his first experience of the horrific injuries caused by firearms. It was here that he discovered that cauterization was not necessary – soldiers with gunshot wounds could be treated more humanely with better results. He presented his new approach in *Method of Treating Wounds* in 1545. Paré went on to become the greatest surgeon of the Renaissance, raising the profile of surgery by becoming a counsellor of state and royal surgeon to four kings of France. He also developed tools and techniques for removing arrowheads and bullets, greatly reducing the need for amputation after traumatic injury in battle. Throughout his life he disdained the theoretical surgical knowledge propounded by those who had studied ancient texts rather than practised surgery. He declared that surgery is 'learnt with the hand and eye'. In 1575, he published a book of nearly 1,000 pages, which summarized the surgical knowledge he had gained from his time in practice.

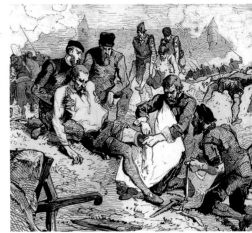

Ambroise Paré working as an army surgeon with an amputation patient. He is said to have declared, 'I dressed him, and God cured him'

He discovered that the wounds of his experimental patients had healed better and with less pain than those he had cauterized.

KNOTS AND KNIVES

A more humane method of staunching bleeding than cauterization was ligaturing (tying off) the blood vessels. Of course, this cannot have been easy with a conscious patient who was doubtless writhing around in great pain. The first mention of ligaturing blood vessels was made by Celsus in the 1st century AD. Then in the 7th century, Paul of Aegina described tying a ligature around a varicose vein before removing it (see p.137). The Arab surgeon Abulcasis, in around AD1000, also recommended methods of ligaturing vessels, as did Paré in the 16th century. Ligatures often introduced infection, though, and this made them far from safe.

From the beginning of the 19th century, research into the efficacy of ligatures led

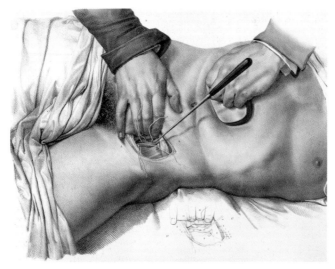

A surgeon applying a ligature to an artery

result with little or no physical contact with the wound.

STITCHES AND SUTURES

Stopping the bleeding is a good start, but the edges of a wound must be held together while the wound heals. Early and non-urbanized societies have often used thorns, gums and resins as sutures, or have bound wounds tightly with bark, leaves or parchment to hold them closed. Although people have used needles for around 20,000 years, they are not thought to have been used for stitching the edges of wounds until around 3000BC, in ancient Egypt. The Egyptians used fibres from plants, hair, wool and animal tendons for suturing. They also used silver wire to clamp wounds. The oldest surviving suture dates from around 1100BC. It was found on the stomach of a mummy.

Indian surgeons also used hair, flax and hemp but they added a bizarre alternative – Bengal ants. Susruta (6th century BC) described a procedure in which Indian

to new developments. One method used forceps to crush the walls of the blood vessel together so that they immediately sealed. Some time before 1812, the Italian Paolo Assalini developed an artery forcep which could be applied with one hand and was spring controlled. Torsion of the arteries was added in 1829. The torsion method is sometimes used alone with smaller vessels: the twisted vessel holds itself closed effectively.

Following the development of asepsis and anaesthesia ligatures became safe. With the patient anaesthetized the surgeon had time to lift and tie each blood vessel before cutting it, minimizing blood loss during surgery. This is a slow process, though, and cauterization continued to be used for smaller blood vessels. More recently, red-hot irons have been replaced by more advanced technology. Cauterization by ultrasound, electric current or laser produces a completely clean and painless

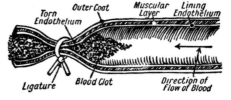

A cross-section through a blood vessel sealed with a ligature shows how it staunches the bleeding in a less painful way than cauterization

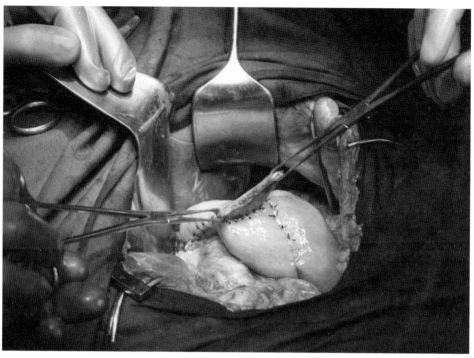

Surgeons applying sutures after surgery on the stomach

surgeons used wood ants to suture internal wounds when they were dealing with abdominal injuries. The surgeon held the edges of the wound together and then applied a large black ant, so that it bit through both sides. He then snapped off the body of the ant, leaving the head to secure the lips of the wound. The intestines were pushed back into the abdomen and the external wound was stitched in the usual way. Other societies, including some in Africa and South America, have also used ants and beetles in this way to suture many types of wounds.

At the time of Hippocrates (c.460–c.375BC) the ancient Greeks used sutures of animal tendon for external wounds and gold wire for bone sutures.

Later on, the ancient Romans used threads of linen, wool and silk, together with human hair and metal clips, to seal wounds. Sutures made of animal gut (chorda) were first described by Galen (AD129–c.216), though they were also used by Indian surgeons. They were probably the first sutures that could be absorbed by the body. Absorbable sutures can be used on internal injuries because they will slowly disappear when the wound has healed.

Arab surgeons such as Rhazes (865–925) and Avicenna (c.980–1037) used material taken from lute strings for both sutures and ligatures. Abulcasis (c.936–1013) gave a detailed description of suture techniques for abdominal wounds as well as for flesh wounds. He used curved and straight needles made of bronze or bone and his suture materials included chorda, hemp, animal fibres, tendon and hair. He used twine or silk as a ligature for blood vessels. The same materials were used in Europe after the opening of the medical schools, with camel hair and camel tendons being added to the list of suitable materials. There was little change in suture materials over the following centuries, though animal materials came to include arteries, nerves and strips of muscle as well as the already common tendons, hair and catgut (any gut used for stringed musical instruments).

Joseph Lister was the first surgeon to sterilize sutures. Carbolic catgut became the first modern suture material in 1860. He introduced chromic catgut, the first suture material specifically developed for surgical use, in 1881. The 1930s saw the first synthetic suture material – a product of the newly emerging chemical industry. In 1931, the first absorbable synthetic suture was introduced, based on polyvinyl alcohol. Many countries abandoned catgut sutures in 2001, because of the danger of Creutzfeldt-Jakob Disease. By then, catgut had been in use for nearly 2,000 years.

THE SURGEON EMBROIDERER

Stitching wounds and even large internal organs does not require the finest of sewing techniques. However, in 1894 the French president Marie-François-Sadi Carnot bled to death after being wounded by an assassin. If the attending surgeons had been able to stitch his severed portal vein he would have lived – but stitching blood vessels is a very different matter from stitching flesh. The event inspired French surgeon Alexis Carrel

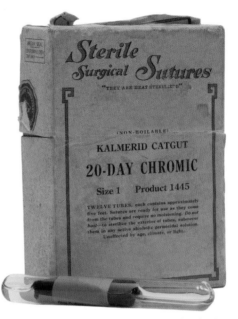

An early pack of chromic catgut, designed to dissolve in 20 days

(1873–1944) to improve things. He had first learned stitching from his mother, but now he took lessons from one of the finest embroiderers in France, Madame Leroidier of Lyons. He first practised on paper, using the finest needles. When he could stitch so finely that the stitches could not be seen on either side, he progressed to animal tissue. Carrel developed a technique of turning back the ends of blood vessels like a cuff, then stitching them end to end so that the blood came into contact with nothing except the interior of the blood vessel. He used paraffin jelly to coat his instruments, needles and threads to prevent clotting and used aseptic techniques to prevent infection. Carrel's work lay behind the microsurgery techniques that are now used in transplant surgery.

ALEXIS CARREL (1873–1944)

Alexis Carrel was born in Lyons, France. His father was a businessman, who died while his son was still very young. Carrel studied medicine in France, where he carried out his early work on stitching blood vessels. He then moved to the United States in 1904, where he began experimenting with transplants. In 1908, he displayed a dog that had lived for 17 months with a transplanted kidney. Carrel won the Nobel Prize in 1912 'in recognition of his work on vascular suture and the transplantation of blood-vessels and organs'.

During the First World War Carrel served as a medical officer with the French army. Working with Englishman Henry Drysdale Dakin, he developed the Carrel-Dakin method of treating war wounds. This consisted of cutting out all of the affected flesh and constantly irrigating the wound with a solution that contained sodium hypochlorite, which was much more effective than earlier bactericides. Wounds sustained in trench warfare were usually infected, because the soil of the French and the Belgian farms had been fertilized with manure for centuries. The Carrel-Dakin method reduced fatal infection from 60 per cent to zero.

In 1935, back in the United States, Carrel worked with the famous aviator Charles Lindbergh to create a machine for providing a sterile respiratory system for transplant organs. He also carried out an experiment to keep cells alive and multiplying outside the body, using heart cells from a chick embryo. He reported keeping the cells alive for 28 years, with the line only dying because of a technician's error. However, it is likely that either error or fraud led to this result because cell lines usually die after around 50 generations. Carrel's laboratory held a birthday party for the chick cells each year on 17 January.

But it was not all grand and heroic. Carrel was a eugenicist and he collaborated with the Vichy government in Nazi-occupied France during the Second World War. Had he not died of a heart attack in 1944, he might have faced a trial for war crimes.

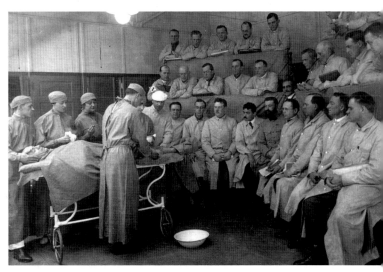

Alexis Carrel giving a demonstration of the Carrel-Dakin method of treating war wounds to French surgeons

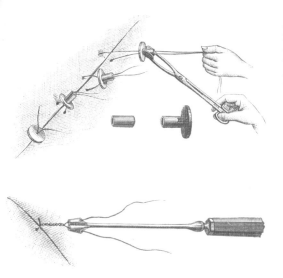

Different methods of applying sutures. To avoid infection, a suture must not allow external fluids to penetrate

The watershed

The twin discoveries of anaesthesia and antisepsis revolutionized surgery. With an inert patient on the table, surgeons were free to develop skills and techniques that took time. Operations without anaesthetic had been traumatic for the surgeon as well as the patient. All this was ended by the 'Yankee dodge' of anaesthesia, while the chances of survival were massively increased by the adoption of antisepsis. In the following 150 years, surgery advanced more than in the preceding 5,000 years.

PRIMITIVE PAINKILLERS

Surgeons had always tried to dull the pain for their patients. Not only was it humane, it was also practical – operating on a writhing, screaming patient was difficult. Alcohol and narcotic drugs, including poppy and marijuana-based concoctions, have been used for millennia, though with mixed success. In the Middle Ages, European surgeons used opium, mandragora (mandrake) or alcohol to deaden pain. Guy de Chauliac (physician to three popes) described a device for delivering some kind of narcotic inhalation to patients, though the details are lost.

There are a number of accounts testifying to the limited effect of alcohol and other painkillers on victims of early surgery. Often, the difficulty of dealing with a drunk or drugged patient led the surgeon to

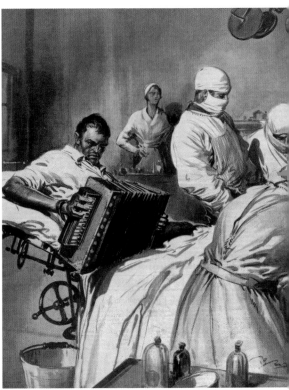

All in the mind: Italian musician Guglielmo Bonfoco refused anaesthetics during his leg amputation, but insisted he be allowed to play his accordian

forgo the painkillers anyway. The accounts of how to hold or tie down a patient are chilling indicators that the pain remained as searing as we would expect. John Woodall called for five assistants when severing a limb, and cutting for the stone required the patient to be securely tied. His or her struggling could have made the operation impossible otherwise.

THE 'YANKEE DODGE'

Dentists must have frequently wrestled with patients who would not keep still, so it is perhaps not surprising that anaesthesia had its beginnings in the dental profession.

The effects of nitrous oxide – laughing gas – were discovered by Joseph Priestley in 1772, and in 1800 Humphry Davy suggested that it might be possible to use the gas during surgery. He did not do it, however – he simply used it to amuse himself, becoming addicted in the process. The English surgeon Henry Hill Hickman did use nitrous oxide as an anaesthetic, but when he published his results in 1824 no one took much notice. Instead, it was used as a recreational drug at parties.

Nitrous oxide was not to be the anaesthetic that made the breakthrough. The real turning point came with William Morton, a dentist, who experimented with ether at the suggestion of a chemist, Charles Jackson. After first trying it on dogs, Morton completed the

Humphry Davy's idea to use nitrous oxide in surgery was disregarded at the time

first painless tooth extraction on a human patient. He published the news in the *Boston Daily Journal*. In 1846 he used ether while he removed a neck tumour (which seems an odd thing for a dentist to be doing) and within two months it was being used in London.

Ether was not ideal because it caused bronchial irritation and it smelled horrible. In Scotland, the obstetrician Sir James Simpson experimented with alternatives and hit upon chloroform in 1847. There was initial resistance – the Church complained that his invention was unchristian because the Book of Genesis had declared that it was God's will that women should bring forth children in pain. Also, a group of American doctors said it was unnatural. Uncowed, Simpson told the Church that God had apparently anaesthetized Adam when removing his rib. He then asked the American doctors if they eschewed the unnatural train when taking long journeys. The royal seal of approval was given when Queen Victoria requested chloroform for the delivery of Prince Leopold, her eighth child, in 1853 – after that, anaesthesia

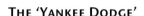

Queen Victoria's use of chloroform during childbirth was a public endorsement of the use of anaesthesia

became immediately acceptable. It was administered to her by John Snow – the man who was destined to confirm the link between cholera and polluted water.

As well as putting the patient to sleep and beyond the reach of pain, anaesthesia relaxes the muscles, making the surgeon's job much easier. But there were problems with early anaesthetics. Chloroform can cause liver damage and even heart failure, while nitrous oxide mixed with oxygen is not powerful enough. Some other gases were tried but they were inflammable, which proved problematic once hospitals began usingprimitive electrical equipment that was prone to sparking.

Intravenous anaesthesia was first developed by Pierre Oré in France in 1874. It became generally used after 1902 when Emil Fischer developed barbital (also known as Veronal), the first commercial barbiturate. Then cocaine was used as a topical anaesthetic in eye surgery and dentistry after being pioneered by Karl Koller in 1884 (following the observation by his friend and colleague, Sigmund Freud, that it numbed pain). Safer drugs, similar to cocaine, are still in use. The injection of cocaine directly into the spine to numb the lower body was first carried out in 1898. It was the precursor of modern epidural anaesthesia, which is commonly used in childbirth.

Antisepsis

Even if operations could be carried out painlessly, they still remained unsafe until the discovery of antiseptics. While Semmelweis' discoveries in Vienna (see p.62)

NOT OUT

Alternatives to chemical painkillers and anaesthesia have included hypnosis, acupuncture and the use of an electric current. Hypnosis and acupuncture have long been used in eastern medicine. In the first half of the 19th century western surgeons, too, began to explore hypnosis. The Scottish surgeon James Braid put patients to sleep by making them stare at a bright object. John Elliotson went a stage further by using hypnosis in operations, publishing his findings in 1843. He was followed in 1845 by James Esdaile, who carried out operations on 261 Hindi prisoners in a Bengali jail, using hypnotism as the only narcotic. When he tried the same thing in his native Scotland it was less successful – whether for cultural or physiological reasons is not clear. In recent years, the use of hypnosis and acupuncture has become popular among western patients who are drawn to complementary therapies.

Another popular alternative to pharmacological analgesia is Transcutaneous Electrical Nerve Stimulation (TENS), which was developed in 1967 by Patrick Wall (who also developed modern epidural anaesthesia). A TENS machine delivers an electric current through electrodes placed on the skin, giving a degree of pain relief during childbirth and to people suffering chronic pain.

James Braid was a pioneer of hypnotism in the West

went largely unheeded, the work of Joseph Lister (1826–1912) in Britain had a revolutionary effect. Since Louis Pasteur had discovered that micro-organisms could cause disease, there was at last an explanation for patients becoming infected and dying after surgery. Lister already suspected that some kind of airborne dust was causing sepsis. He had seen carbolic acid being used to treat foul-smelling sewage, so he began to carry out operations under a fine spray of the substance, which proved to be a strong antiseptic. Levels of infection immediately fell. Lister had recorded a death rate of around 45 to 50 per cent amongst his amputation patients between 1861 and 1865, but by 1869 (using antisepsis) the death rate had fallen to 15 per cent.

During the Franco-Prussian war, the surgeons of the Prussian army experimented further with antisepsis and there were fewer deaths among war casualties as a result. However, Lister's work was little recognized outside Scotland and Prussia until he took the chair of surgery at King's College, London, in 1877. At last he had the chance to make the world take notice. In the year of his appointment, he advertised that he was going to wire a fractured patella (kneecap) under antiseptic conditions. The operation was rarely performed because it involved converting a simple fracture into a compound fracture, which usually became infected and killed the patient. The success of his operation at last convinced Britain and America that antisepsis was the way forward.

Remaking the body

The most significant change in surgery has been the move from removing damaged parts to attempting to repair or replace them. The opportunity to spend longer on an operation has made this possible – the surgeon no longer has to get in and out as quickly as possible before the patient dies of shock. Two areas in which repairing and replacing have had the most impact are reconstructive surgery and transplants.

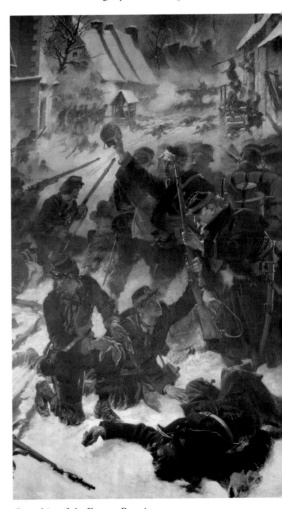

Casualties of the Franco-Prussian war were among the first to benefit from antiseptic wound treatment following Joseph Lister's research

FACING THE WORLD WITH PLASTIC SURGERY

Reconstructive surgery depends heavily on skin grafts, so it could not be developed significantly until grafting had been perfected. Experiments with skin-grafting had been conducted well before the 20th century, though. As we have seen, the Indian surgeon Susruta reconstructed noses, earlobes and cleft lips as early as the 6th century BC, and the Italian Gaspare Tagliacozzi practised rhinoplasty in the 16th century (see p.134). News of the Indian method of nose reconstruction reached Europe in 1794, and a skin graft on a sheep followed in 1804. In 1823, Christian Bünger carried out the first successful full-thickness skin graft in Europe by taking skin from a patient's thigh and grafting it on to a reconstructed nose. (Previous nose reconstructions had required the skin to be attached by a flap to its original site until the graft had taken.) The Swiss doctor Jacques Reverdin discovered that grafts were more successful if just a layer of skin was used, rather than the full thickness. He used skin grafts to treat ulcers and burns in 1869 and he was the first surgeon to attempt grafting between

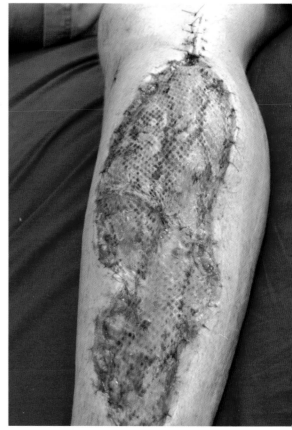

A fasciotomy operation, in which the leg has been cut to relieve internal pressure. A skin graft helps to heal the wound

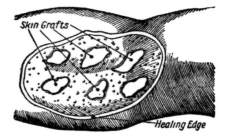

Skin grafts over an open wound aid the healing process, as the patient does not need to wait for skin to grow from the edges

Swiss surgeon Jacques Louis Reverdin

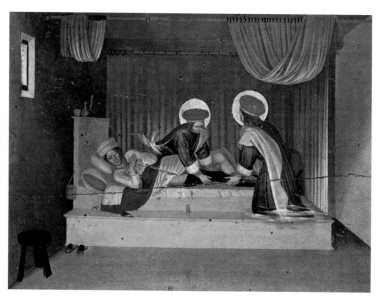

Legend tells us that saints Cosmas and Damien transplanted a leg from a Moor to a white Christian

people. In 1881, skin from a corpse was used for the first time in a temporary graft. The patient was suffering severe burns from a singularly unlucky accident: he had been leaning against a metal door which had been struck by lightning.

If anaesthesia and antisepsis made plastic surgery possible, the First World War made it essential. The demands placed on the medical profession by the ravages of the First World War prompted more ambitious reconstructive surgery. Soldiers with shattered faces confronted a wrecked life until surgeon Harold Gillies stepped into the picture. By using pioneering techniques Gillies and his team restored (with varying degrees of success) the faces of thousands of men who had been injured in the First World War. Gillies would spend at least an hour visualizing each reconstruction. On some occasions he made sketches, which he cut up and moved around, while at other times he moulded the new face in wax. His main

technique, though, was to create a plaster model of the patient's new face. In Germany, at about the same time, Jacques Joseph carried out similar reconstructive work on badly disfigured German soldiers. He believed that cosmetic surgery, while not a physical necessity, was worth the health risk it posed because of its positive psychological impact. He came to be considered the first plastic surgeon in Europe.

Gillies' distant cousin, Archibald McIndoe, developed new techniques for reconstructing badly burned faces and hands in the Second World War. McIndoe went beyond plastic surgery by concerning himself with the social reintegration and psychological reconstruction of his badly damaged patients. After he was appointed plastic surgeon to the Royal Air Force he ran a hospital and rehabilitation unit in East Grinstead, which was unique in its relaxed and humane treatment of horribly mutilated airmen.

HAROLD GILLIES (1882–1960)

Born in New Zealand, Gillies moved to Britain to study medicine at Cambridge University. At the start of the First World War, he was posted with the army medical corps to Belgium where he met Bob Roberts, a dentist who was keen on exploring jaw reconstruction surgery, and Auguste Valadier, a specialist in jaw wounds. When he returned to England, Gillies persuaded the army to open a unit for reconstructive facial surgery. He and his team performed over 11,000 operations on 5,000 injured soldiers, most of whom had been shot in the face. He worked in private practice between the wars and then became a plastic surgery consultant to the armed forces during the Second World War. When a distant cousin, Archibald McIndoe, arrived in London to discover that the job he had been promised did not exist, Gillies took him under his wing. They formed the greatest surgical partnership of the 20th century. Gillies taught McIndoe to become as great a plastic surgeon as he was himself. In 1946 Gillies and McIndoe pioneered one of the first gender reassignment operations.

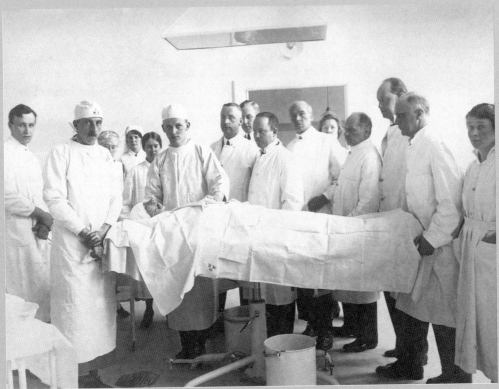

Harold Gillies attends a Danish sailor in the operating theatre of the Navy Hospital, Copenhagen, in 1924. The patient was injured in an explosion on a warship

New Organs for Old

Transplant surgery had been attempted many centuries before it could ever have been successful. The very first experiments with transplants were an unmitigated failure. Before organ transplants could be tackled with any hope of success, medical science needed to discover and understand blood groups (see p.31), develop techniques for stitching blood vessels, muscles and nerves (see p.154) and tackle the problem of rejection by the immune system.

Apart from the skin grafts that were part of the nose reconstruction surgery described by Susruta, the earliest reported tissue transplant was a bone graft. Surgeon Job van Meekeren apparently used a portion of bone from a dog's cranium to patch the skull of a man in either 1668 or 1682. The report relating to 1682 claims that the man was a Russian aristocrat and that the graft later had to be removed because he was threatened with excommunication by the Church. There appear to have been no more tissue transplants until 1880, when a corneal transplant was attempted, apparently without success. The Austrian ophthalmologist Edward Zirm carried out a similar operation successfully in 1905.

Two crucial developments made further progress possible. The first was Austrian ·Karl Landsteiner's discovery of different blood groups in 1900, and the second was Alexis Carrel's fine stitching technique. These developments enabled early experiments in kidney transplants using kidneys from animals. The kidneys were attached to blood vessels in various parts of the human body, but they only ever functioned for very short periods. In 1936,

the Russian surgeon Yuriy Voronoy carried out the first human-to-human kidney transplant on a 26-year-old woman, but the organ failed after two days. After several further unsuccessful attempts, the first true success came in 1954 when American surgeon Joseph E. Murray transplanted a kidney between identical twins and the kidney functioned for several years. Murray shared the Nobel Prize for Medicine in 1990.

From Kidneys to Faces

Reliable, successful transplants were made possible when the problem of tissue graft rejection was solved. One of the pioneers in this field was the British researcher Sir Peter Medawar who discovered during the 1940s and 1950s that organ grafts were rejected because of an immune system response. He shared a Nobel Prize in 1960 for his work.

This knowledge paved the way for the discovery of immunosuppressant drugs, which prevented the white blood cells of the recipient from attacking the donated tissue. This was the breakthrough point for transplant surgery. The first successful transplant from a dead donor followed in 1962 – the kidney recipient lived for 21 months. Transplants came thick and fast after this: liver (1963); lung (1963); pancreas (1966); and – the Holy Grail of transplant surgery – heart (1967). Not all of these transplants were successful: the recipients only survived for a few days in some cases. Even so, the viability of the procedure was proven. The successes became more frequent as the surgeons gained experience and the immunosuppressant drugs improved. The postoperative survival

THE FIRST HEART TRANSPLANT

The first heart transplant operation was carried out by the South African surgeon Christiaan Barnard in 1967. His patient was Louis Washkansky, a a 54-year-old grocer with congestive heart failure. Barnard performed the first South African kidney transplant in 1959, but he did not attempt a human heart transplant until he had practised on over 50 dogs. Washkansky received the heart of a young woman, Denise Darvall, who had been killed in a road accident. He lived for only 18 days before dying of pneumonia, a consequence of the immunosuppressant drugs he was taking.

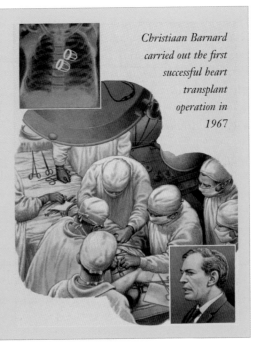

Christiaan Barnard carried out the first successful heart transplant operation in 1967

period stretched out to weeks, then months and finally years. At the same time, a growing variety of organs and tissues began to be transplanted successfully. In 1973 the first successful bone marrow transplant from an unrelated donor was carried out in New York and 1983 saw the first successful single lung transplant – the patient survived for more than six years. Then in 1988 the first sciatic nerve transplant enabled a 9-year-old boy to walk again after an accident.

In 1983, organ transplantation was revolutionized when cyclosporin was isolated from a fungus growing in Norwegian soil. Transplant procedures that had previously seen a high failure rate (including heart transplants) were immediately made viable by this immunosuppressant drug.

Other body parts, such as hands, feet and even faces, became candidates for transplant surgery as microsurgery techniques improved to the point at which small blood vessels and nerves could be reconnected. The first hand transplant was carried out in France in 1998, but it was reversed in 2001 when the recipient insisted that the transplanted hand be removed. Other hand transplants have been more successful. The

> *For a dying person, a transplant is not a difficult decision. If a lion chases you to a river filled with crocodiles, you will leap into the water convinced you have a chance to swim to the other side. But you would never accept such odds if there were no lion.*
>
> Christiaan Barnard

first face transplant patient was French woman Isabelle Dinoir, who lost her nose, lips and chin in an attack by a savage dog. The transplant, which was performed in 2005, laid to rest fears that a transplanted face would look too much like the donor for people to be comfortable with it.

HELPING HANDS – AND FEET

Long before transplants appeared on the scene, missing or damaged body parts were repaired or replaced using a variety of materials and techniques. Prosthetic limbs are one of the oldest forms of medical technology and were one of the earliest ways of supplying some of the function of a missing or damaged part. For instance, an Egyptian mummy has been found with a prosthetic toe. In around 484BC, Herodotus told of a captured Persian soldier called Hegesistratus who had escaped by cutting through his chained foot, and later replaced

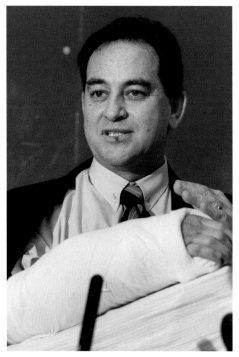

The world's first hand transplant patient, Clint Hallam, later had the hand removed by surgeons

SURGEON AS SUSHI CHEF

The shortage of organs for transplant surgery is a worldwide problem which has spawned a gruesome, illegal market. Tales of people murdered for their organs are hard to verify, but witnesses in China have testified to the harvesting of organs from executed criminals. A Chinese medic who had gone to live in the United States, where he worked as a sushi chef, furnished a graphic account of organ collection in his home country. Blood samples were taken from condemned prisoners in order to match them to the recipients of their organs. They were then injected with anti-coagulants before execution. Organs were removed in the back of a moving ambulance on the journey between the execution ground and the crematorium. Skin for grafting was stripped from the body at the same time. Sometimes the criminals were not even dead when their organs were taken – the Chinese medic turned chef told US Congressional investigators that he had seen kidneys removed from victims who were still breathing. Surgeons in China paid the equivalent of US$45 for a criminal's body and the hospitals then charged foreign customers up to US$50,000 for a kidney transplant.

MONKEYING AROUND WITH THE LIBIDO

Serge Voronoff (1866–1951) was a Russian surgeon who settled in France and studied under Alexis Carrel. Observing the effects of castration on young boys in Egypt between 1896 and 1910, he decided that something in the testicles might prevent ageing. He experimented with transplanting testicles between animals, then he tried taking them from executed criminals and putting them into wealthy clients. When he ran out of criminals he moved on to primates (chimpanzees and baboons). In 1920 he carried out his first operation to implant slices of monkey testicle into the scrotum of a Frenchman. By 1923, more than 700 surgeons had applauded his success in apparently rejuvenating old men. Thousands of the operations were carried out worldwide, though a shortage of monkeys threatened the procedure. A less flamboyant method was the so-called Steinach operation, which was no more than vasectomy. The Irish poet W.B. Yeats was convinced that the operation gave him renewed sexual vigour.

the lost part with a wooden prosthesis. When a Roman general, Marcus Sergius, lost a hand in the Punic War he had an iron one made so that he could hold his shield and return to the field of battle. Survivors of trephination and skull injuries in pre-Columbian South America sometimes had prosthetic implants made of gourd skin and gold sheet to fill in the gaps where bone was missing. Knights in the Middle Ages constantly ran the risk of losing a limb. Victims often had a fake arm produced by their armourers – as much to hide the loss of an arm (an embarrassing indicator of past failure) as to provide any useful function. These early prosthetics could do little more than provide a prop (in the case of a leg) or a primitive claw or hook (in the case of a hand). Sometimes they were just added to improve the appearance of the patient – glass eyes, in particular, were used for cosmetic reasons rather than for function.

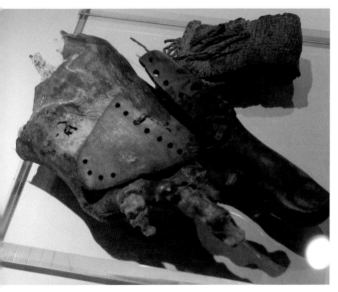

A wooden toe found on an Egyptian mummy reveals just how long prosthetic parts have existed

In around 1530 Ambroise Paré began to design more

functional prosthetics for his amputation patients. These included articulated hands made of metal and leather with jointed, hinged fingers, and legs with locking knee joints. Then in 1696 the Dutch surgeon Pieter Verduyn produced a lower-leg prosthesis with hinges and a leather cuff for attaching it to the body. By 1800 prosthetics were rapidly improving – artificial tendons were incorporated into the 'Anglesey leg' (made for the Marquess of Anglesey), which made the toe lift when the knee was bent. Twelve years later an artificial arm controlled by the opposite shoulder was developed, and the first artificial limb to move through muscle contraction appeared in 1898.

The invention of plastics and robotics has paved the way to great developments in appearance and functionality. Today's prosthetic limbs look lifelike, and may be custom-made to match the patient's own original limb very closely. A robotic prosthetic limb combines sensors and processors with a small motor which drives the movement of the limb. Some sensors pick up electrical signals from the nerves and muscles of the remaining tissue, while others respond to stimuli from the environment (such as pressure). A microprocessor in the controller of the limb calculates the necessary movement and controls the action of the prosthesis.

Ongoing research into assisted vision systems hopes to produce functional replacement eyes, too. Implants with light sensitive cells will respond to light falling on them to send an electrical signal through the optic nerve to the brain, producing a serviceable image. The resulting 'bionic'

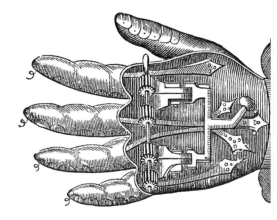

An articulated prosthetic hand designed by Ambroise Paré around 1530

eye should give rudimentary vision to some blind people.

HIPS AND HEARTS

Until the late 19th century, joints that had been broken or damaged by arthritis, tuberculosis, syphilis and other conditions could be treated only by amputation or surgery. During early hip surgery the bones were removed or trimmed in order to encourage soft tissue growth. Although a degree of functionality was sometimes achieved, the procedure came with a relatively low survival rate (around 50 per cent). In an attempt to reduce friction, surgeons attached a variety of materials to the trimmed hip joint, including gold foil and pig's bladder. Even so, patients lost mobility in the joint within a few years.

The first feasible replacement hip joint appeared in 1891, when German surgeon Themistocles Gluck made an ivory ball and socket joint. Nickel-plated screws fixed it to the bone that remained after surgery. During the course of the 20th century, a

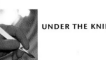
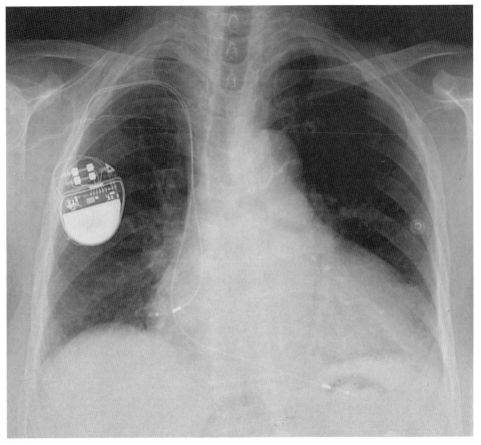

An artificial pacemaker implanted into a patient's chest is clearly visible in a radiograph. Modern pacemakers now allow the cardiologist to select the optimum pace rate for the individual patient

number of materials have been used as prosthetic ends for the femur, including rubber, glass, Bakelite and the dental material Vitallium. In 1960 the Burmese surgeon San Baw began using ivory replacement joints at Mandalay General Hospital, Burma; they were the first generally successful artificial hip joints. The modern replacement hip uses titanium stainless steel components cemented to the patient's bone. It was developed in England during the 1960s by Sir John Charnley.

One of the most widely used medical replacements is the heart pacemaker, which takes over the role of the heart's natural pacemaker cells in the sinoatial node, by regulating the heartbeat when required. The English surgeon W.H. Walshe suggested using electric impulses to restart the heart in 1862 (defibrillation), but it took almost another century before the first pacemakers appeared. American cardiologist Paul Zoll first tried passing an electrode down the oesophagus of a patient but this did not work, so in 1952 he developed an external pacemaker that sent electric shocks to the heart through the chest. Although the shocks were painful, the machine kept a patient alive for two days until his own heart took over. The external pacemaker was large and had to be connected to a mains electricity supply, but until the development of transistors and small batteries an internal model was not feasible. That changed in 1958 when Rune Elmqvist and Åke Senning in Sweden made a pacemaker that could be implanted in the chest. Later developments in technology led to pacemakers that could adjust the heartbeat to the patient's level of activity. Others can be reprogrammed using radio and will even transmit information about the patient's health using mobile telephone technology. Many modern pacemakers log information about the patient's condition and this can be downloaded to a hospital computer.

Surgery comes of age

In the ancient world, the doctors who took their orders directly from the gods ranked more highly than the men who cut, with hope and skill but little knowledge, into the hapless patient. As it became acceptable to look inside the dead human body, surgeons were finally able to learn more about the object of their attentions. The profession then divided into those with practical skills and those with a university education. Occasionally some had both. But until the 20th century, surgery was risky and

sometimes terrifying. If the patient did not die from shock, he or she would very likely die of infection. Often the agony of surgery produced little lasting benefit. Then, with the benefit of anaesthetics, antisepsis, antibiotics and immunosuppressant drugs, surgeons began to mend or replace dysfunctional organs instead of simply cutting them out. Since the work of Harold Gillies and Sir Archibald McIndoe it has even become common for people to have elective surgery, such as facelifts or breast reduction, that is often far from necessary.

The surgeons of the future will have less and less contact with the blood and gore that marked their predecessors. Many modern surgical treatments use waves of energy, such as ultrasound and lasers, in place of the knives and saws of earlier times. An increasing number of techniques are carried out by laparoscopy, or keyhole surgery, which requires making one or more small incisions through which procedures can be carried out using endoscopes and tiny tools controlled by surgical robots. Using telesurgery, the surgeon need not even be in the same physical space as the patient. Instead, he or she controls a surgical robot over the internet, using cameras or virtual reality techniques. Nanotechnology offers further possibilities for the future. We may soon be able to send tiny machines into the body to fix it from the inside, controlled remotely and minimally invasive for the patient. It is a far cry from the trephining drill and the dismembering saw.

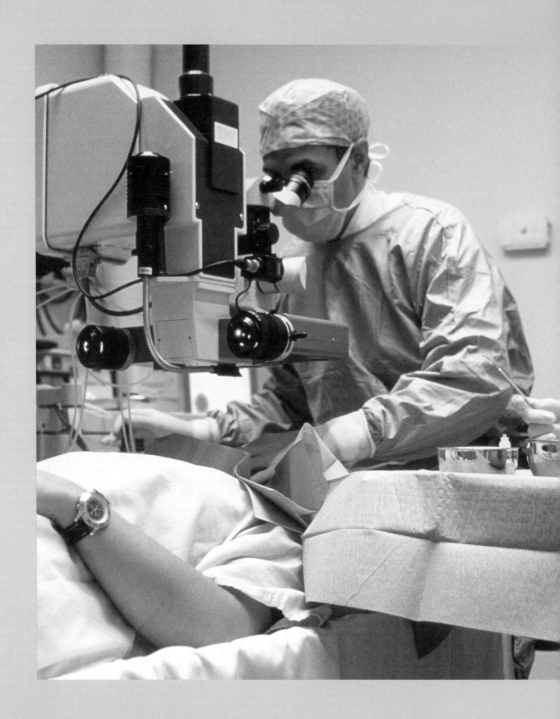

CHAPTER 6

THE LONG ART

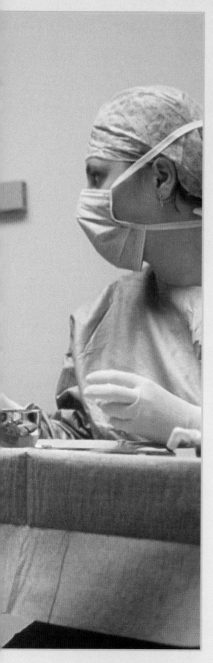

At the dawn of civilization, medicine was a magical art. People had little understanding of how the body worked and how it could go wrong, so an appeal to the gods was perhaps as good a means of obtaining a cure as any other.

As people began to study and think about the body, medicine moved away from magic and religion and, at least in the West, became a science. The professionals that had been entrusted with the care of the body learned practical skills and acquired knowledge that was based on reasoning and observation – even if it was sometimes fairly inaccurate.

Men and, later, women had to undertake training or an apprenticeship before they could practise medicine. Eventually, this formalized into a period of long academic study and supervised clinical practice before someone could work either as a doctor, a nurse, a midwife, a surgeon or other medical specialist.

Every member of the medical team has undergone years of training: each discipline requires expert knowledge

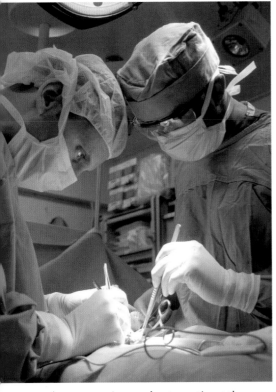

A surgeon carries out a heart operation at the Fitzsimons Army Medical Center

Deities and doctors

The respect and prestige enjoyed by modern doctors pales into insignificance beside the status afforded healers by some ancient cultures. Because illness and recovery were shrouded in mystery, doctors were sometimes elevated to the position of priests or even gods.

Even though medical knowledge is no longer thought to be divinely bestowed, doctors are still revered and respected. Some – like the dashing Christiaan Barnard – became international celebrities.

EARLY DOCTOR-GODS

The Greek god Asclepius and the Egyptian Imhotep (fl.27th century BC) were both physician gods. Renowned as a healer, Imhotep was acclaimed as the originator of Egyptian medicine – he possibly wrote the text that is preserved in the Edwin Smith papyrus. Although the work removes medicine from the realm of magic, Imhotep was made into a demigod 100 years after his

---

IMHOTEP (FL.27TH CENTURY BC)

Imhotep was probably the royal chamberlain (or vizier) to King Netjerikhet (also known as Djoser), who ruled c.2635–2610BC. A formidable polymath, he was commissioned to build the Step Pyramid (the first tomb in Egypt to be built entirely of stone); he was high priest to the sun god Ra at Heliopolis; he was chief carpenter, sculptor and vase maker; and he was also the first physician to be known by name. Credited with inventing the papyrus scroll, he became the patron spirit of scribes, who often poured out a libation to him before beginning work. Imhotep's tomb has never been found.

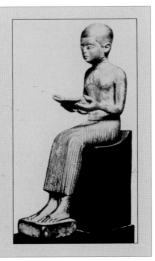

A statue of the Egyptian doctor-god Imhotep

death. He was raised to full deity status around 525BC.

In Graeco-Roman times, temples to Imhotep in Memphis and on the island of Philae in the Nile River were popular venues for temple sleep.

In ancient Greece, Imhotep became associated with Asclepius, the Greek god of medicine. According to mythology Asclepius was the son of Apollo, who had been taught medicine by the centaur Chiron. However, a real man may lie behind the legend.

According to Homer's *Iliad*, Asclepius was a skilful physician and the father of two doctors called Machaon and Podalirius. Sufferers took to sleeping in his temple at Epidaurus, hoping for a miraculous cure or a sign. His cult spread to Rome in 293BC, where he was worshipped as Aesculapius (the Latinized form of his name). The medical symbol of a snake twined around a staff is taken from traditional images of Asclepius.

NOT GODS, BUT STILL PRETTY GOOD

The towering medical figures of the classical world were Hippocrates, Celsus and Galen. The influence they exerted over the ensuing 2,000 years both stifled and inspired later physicians.

Hippocrates (c.460–c.375BC) was never honoured as a god, but he was still revered as a great physician and teacher of medicine for two millennia. Along with Hippocrates, the later Graeco-Roman physician Galen (AD129–c.216) (see p.22) dominated medicine until the 18th century.

Galen's extensive writings and the Hippocratic Corpus together comprise the entire body of medical achievement in Greek antiquity.

Many of Galen's works were saved from obscurity during the Dark Ages when they were translated into Arabic in the 9th century. At the same time they became the foundations on which Arab medicine was built.

From the 11th century onwards these Arabic texts began to be translated into Latin and Galen's works soon came to dominate teaching in the medieval European medical schools.

Ironically, Galen's own injunction to observe and experiment led to the discovery of errors in his works and his eventual dethronement as the ultimate authority.

Aulus Cornelius Celsus (c.25BC–c.50AD) also loomed large in the medieval medical schools. Although he was apparently not famous

Asclepius complete with entwined serpent and stick

during his lifetime, he became hugely influential nearly 1,500 years later, when his work was rediscovered in 1426.

It is thought that he wrote a large encyclopedia, but only the volume on medicine, *De medicina*, has survived. In 1478 it became one of the first medical works to be published after the development of printing in the West. Celsus was probably not a doctor himself (the lost volumes of his work treated such diverse subjects as rhetoric, law, agriculture, philosophy and military strategy), but he minutely recorded the advanced state of medicine in 1st-century Rome. He explains how to ligature blood vessels; rebuild noses, lips and ears; remove bladder stones; and splint broken bones – he also gives accounts of heart disease and insanity. His descriptions of medical tools exactly match instruments that were found at Pompeii, the site of the eruption of Vesuvius in AD79.

Celsus was held in such high regard that the 16th-century Swiss doctor Theophrastus Bombastus von Hohenheim (1493–1541) (see p.115) took the name Paracelsus ('equal to or greater than Celsus'), trading on his reputation but claiming to be better than him.

The mighty fallen

With the coming of the Renaissance and the resurgence of anatomy, people began to discover errors in the work of the great classical authorities. William Harvey revealed the mistakes in Galen's model of the heart and the blood and Andreas Vesalius announced that Galen's dependence on animal anatomy had led him to false conclusions.

Great doctors have not always been revered. Innovators such as Harvey and Vesalius were at first derided or even ridiculed. Some did not live to see their revolutionary ideas taken up by mainstream medicine, and there are countless examples of breakthroughs that languished for years before their value was recognized. In Vienna, Ignaz Semmelweis (1818–65) (see p.62) ended up in a madhouse, driven over the edge by the medical profession's refusal to adopt the hygiene measures he knew would save hundreds of lives. Henry Hill Hickman (1800–30) failed to persuade anyone to take his pioneering anaesthesia experiments seriously, and John Snow (1813–58) died before the biological cause of cholera was recognized by his profession.

Before man and god

Being a surgeon or a doctor has always carried a lot of responsibility and doing it badly has often had legal consequences.

The earliest surviving legal code was laid out by Hammurabi, King of Babylon (c.1795–1750BC). It is preserved on a stone pillar 2 metres tall (7 feet), which is kept in the Louvre in Paris, France. Not only does it stipulate the price of a surgical operation but it also lists the punishments that an incompetent (or unfortunate) surgeon would have faced.

In Babylon, a freeman would pay five silver shekels for a surgeon to carry out an operation or cure an eye disease, while the charge for curing a slave was only two shekels, paid by the slave's owner. If the surgeon did it wrong, and his mistake cost the patient his life or his sight, the surgeon's hands were cut off. Similarly, if the surgeon

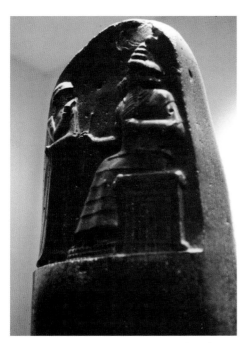

King Hammurabi depicted on the stone that also records his legal code

doctors in many western nations must follow. Strict guidance on the proper behaviour of a good doctor is offered, not only in the oath itself but also in the Hippocratic writings:

For the physician it is undoubtedly an important recommendation to be of good appearance and well-fed, since people take the view that those who do not know how to look after their own bodies are in no position to look after those of others. He must know how and when to be silent, and to live an ordered life, as this greatly enhances his reputation. His bearing must be that of an honest man, for this he must be towards all honest people, and kindly and understanding. He must not act impulsively or hastily, he must look calm, serene and never cross; on the other hand, it does not do for him to be too jolly.

Hippocrates advocates that the doctor should also be clean, and have a good haircut – people did not want a shabby, smelly doctor by their sickbed in the 4th century BC, any more than they do now. Hippocratic doctors conducted house visits, but they also set up a stall or a shop in a public place where patients could call in for a prognosis. Passers-by and any other interested parties could often observe the consultation and even venture an opinion.

Fellow feeling

While illness and surgery have always been traumatic for patients, dealing with affliction has often been an ordeal for doctors and surgeons, too. For people with the compassionate nature that drives them

killed a patient when lancing an abscess his hands would be forfeit – unless the patient was a slave, in which case the surgeon need only replace the slave with another. It took a brave and confident man to work as a surgeon in ancient Babylon.

Codes of behaviour have long been associated with medical practice. Sumerian doctors were required to follow certain ethical standards in their practices. They were not allowed to prescribe expensive remedies if there was no hope that a patient would recover. Instead they should ease the patient's last days and offer consolation to the family, giving an honest prognosis.

The Hippocratic oath is the most famous code of behaviour for doctors. It still forms the basis of the ethical code that

to practise medicine, impotence in the face of suffering and – worse – the need to inflict suffering exacts a great personal price. The distress experienced by doctors when they are undertaking their duties should not be underestimated. Writing about the plague of Justinian, Procopius (AD499–565) sympathized with the misery suffered by the doctors tending the sick:

And those who were attending them were in a state of constant exhaustion and had a most difficult time of it throughout. For this reason everybody pitied them no less than the sufferers, not because they were threatened by the pestilence in going near it... but they pitied them because of the great hardships which they were undergoing.

Ambroise Paré was moved by the distress that patients felt when confronted by the traditional cauterization of wounds – he was reluctant to carry it out until his colleagues assured him that it was necessary for their survival (see p.150). In Fanny Burney's traumatic account of her surgery for breast cancer (see p.149), one of the most striking elements is her description of the terrible distress of the surgeon who had to inflict such suffering on her:

I then saw my good Dr. Larry, pale nearly as myself, his face streaked with blood, its expression depicting grief, apprehension, & almost horrour.

The practice of Caesarian section similarly aroused a strong feeling of horror in the surgeons who had to perform it, as can be seen from this 18th-century text:

Its sole idea will force the most intrepid to tremble. Judge also what resolution one ought to have to qualify one to open the belly of a living woman making in it an incision about a half a foot long then groping in the cavity of the abdomen, cut like a wound in the body of the matrix [uterus]; then pierce the membranes, and draw out a child through all these apertures. This operation terrifies and affrights the chirurgeon, even when performed after the death of the woman. What horror then should it not excite, when accompanied with the cries of a mother, which we force to suffer with unparallel'd cruelty, and the effusion of a prodigious quantity of blood, which flowing out by the great wounds, may kill her in an instant, while in the hands of the operator?

Pierre Dionis, *A Course of Chirurgical Operations*, 1733, p.87

In the 1639 edition of *The Surgeon's Mate*, John Woodall tells the surgeon to keep the terrible implements of amputation out of sight of his patients. The compassion exhibited towards the poor patient is remarkable, but he also recommends that the surgeon have an eye on his own reputation and the fate of his soul, just in case compassion is not enough. If the surgeon cuts with a cavalier attitude, Woodall warns, he may not only 'be esteemed Butcher-like and hatefull' but 'thou maist answer thy deed both here and in the world to come. For the subject of thy Art is the most precious of Gods creatures.'

THE HIPPOCRATIC OATH

Newly qualified doctors may choose to take the oath, though most medical schools no longer insist on it.

I swear by Apollo the physician, and Asclepius, and Hygieia and Panacea and all the gods and goddesses as my witnesses, that, according to my ability and judgement, I will keep this Oath and this contract:

To hold him who taught me this art equally dear to me as my parents, to be a partner in life with him, and to fulfil his needs when required; to look upon his offspring as equals to my own siblings, and to teach them this art, if they shall wish to learn it, without fee or contract; and that by the set rules, lectures, and every other mode of instruction, I will impart a knowledge of the art to my own sons, and those of my teachers, and to students bound by this contract and having sworn this Oath to the law of medicine, but to no others.

I will use those dietary regimens which will benefit my patients according to my greatest ability and judgement, and I will do no harm or injustice to them.

I will not give a lethal drug to anyone if I am asked, nor will I advise such a plan; and *similarly I will not give a woman a pessary to cause an abortion.*

In purity and according to divine law will I carry out my life and my art.

I will not use the knife, even upon those suffering from stones, but I will leave this to those who are trained in this craft.

Into whatever homes I go, I will enter them for the benefit of the sick, avoiding any voluntary act of impropriety or corruption, including the seduction of women or men, whether they are free men or slaves.

Whatever I see or hear in the lives of my patients, whether in connection with my professional practice or not, which ought not to be spoken of outside, I will keep secret, as considering all such things to be private.

So long as I maintain this Oath faithfully and without corruption, may it be granted to me to partake of life fully and the practice of my art, gaining the respect of all men for all time. However, should I transgress this Oath and violate it, may the opposite be my fate.

Translated by Michael J. North, The US National Library of Medicine

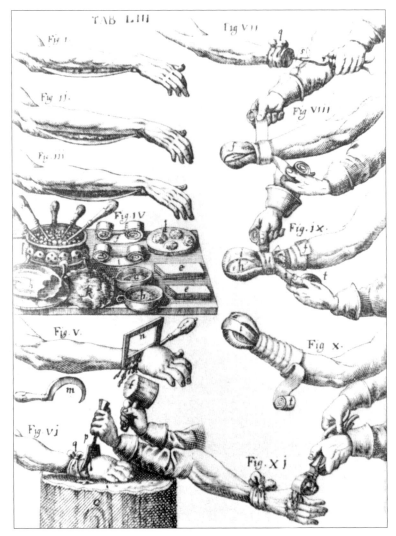

From incision to amputation: a historical artwork of arm surgery from J Scultetus'
Armamentarium Chirurgicum *(1665)*

The art is long...

Most cultures have demanded that proper training of some kind should be undertaken before anyone could practise medicine. The young man (for medicine has usually been a male province) who aspired to medicine first had to learn about the prevailing model of the body and all of the known diseases. Then he had to learn to observe and interpret the signs and symptoms of the patient before finally familiarizing himself with all of the medicines and procedures available. Even in the time of Hippocrates, it took a long time to train as a doctor.

DOCTORS OF DEATH

Although compassion is usually a driving force in people who choose to train as doctors, a few of them have used their knowledge to cause harm instead. Some historians believe that the infamous 19th-century London serial killer Jack the Ripper was a surgeon, on account of the clinically precise dismemberment of the bodies of his victims. The more recent serial killer Harold Shipman used his position as a general practitioner to poison many elderly patients.

However, it is still difficult to comprehend why so many qualified doctors were willing to torture and kill for the Nazis. The most famous of these was Dr Josef Mengele, who was known as 'the angel of death'. Working in the concentration camps, these doctors carried out 'medical experiments' on prisoners, many of them horribly cruel.

It was claimed that these experiments were designed to help the German war effort, by providing information about the human body's reaction to low temperatures or poisonous gases used as a weapon. Other experiments tested new treatments for disease.

Many of these 'experiments' were thinly disguised exercises in torture, though. There has since been debate about whether the results of the experiments can be used by ethical scientists. Tests of the sulpha drugs that were used extensively as antibiotics in and after the Second World War were carried out on 86 prisoners at the Ravensbrück camp. At least five of the test subjects died during the experiments.

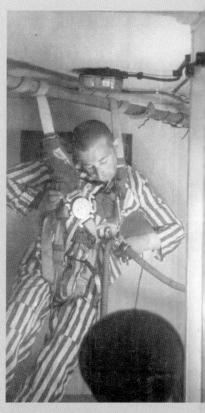

A Jewish prisoner at Dachau concentration camp forced to take part in medical 'experiments' into the effects of high altitude

MEDICAL SCHOOLS

Although Asclepius was supposedly taught medicine by the centaur Chiron, Hippocrates learned his art from mortal teachers – his father and the teachers at the asclepion at Kos. There were differing approaches to medicine in the Ancient Greek medical schools. One of the greatest, the school at Knidos, tended to focus on diseases, while its competitor at Kos looke

at the patient as a whole. This second approach was in accord with Hippocrates' preference for a holistic view, and became the foundation of the Hippocratic medical tradition.

Hippocrates spent much time travelling around Greece and Asia Minor and also teaching at the medical school at Kos. He is said to have taught sitting under a plane tree there, which became famous (see p.18).

179

A possible descendant of that same tree still stands. Kos remained the principal medical school of the Hellenic world for centuries, during which time it carried on teaching the scientific doctrine of Hippocrates. The University of the Aegean is now considering establishing a new medical school at Kos.

The next great medical school of antiquity was founded at Alexandria in Egypt in about 300BC. It attracted the best Greek physicians: Herophilos and Erasistratus both taught there. They were perhaps the first doctors to study anatomy through dissection (see p.21). The school at Alexandria supplied Rome with many of its doctors, including Galen.

When the Hellenic world fell under the rule of first Rome and then Byzantium, progress in medicine diminished in Europe. The focus moved instead to the Middle East. During the 6th century the great medical academy at Jundi Shāhpūr (Gundishapur) in southern Persia came to prominence. It housed both a hospital and a school under the Sassanid emperor Khosrau I (AD531–79). He took in refugee Greek and Nestorian Christian philosophers, many of whom were fleeing persecution by the Byzantines, and engaged them in translating classical medical texts into Persian. Indian and Chinese doctors were also welcomed to the academy so medical texts from Sanskrit and Chinese were translated, too. Teachers at the academy transformed medical education: students worked in the hospital under the eye of the whole medical faculty, rather than being apprenticed to a single doctor. They then had to pass examinations before being allowed to practise. In 638 Persia fell to the Muslim Arab armies. The school still flourished under Arab rule but the Greek texts were now translated into

DOCTOR IN DISGUISE

The writer Gaius Julius Hyginus (c.64BC–AD17), who came from Roman Spain, relates the story of a woman in Egypt called Agnodice who disguised herself as a man in order to learn the practice of medicine. The Athenians, he reports, did not allow women or slaves to train in medicine. As women were ashamed to accept a male attendant during labour, many died in childbirth. Agnodice cut her hair, donned men's clothing, and trained under Herophilos at Alexandria. She then worked as a midwife. Because she was still in disguise, she lifted up her undergarments to show the patient she was really a woman. She became so popular with her female patients that she was called before the Areopagus (court) to answer charges of seducing her patients. Again she raised her clothing to show that she was female. Support for her was such that the Athenians amended the law so that women could train in medicine.

Agnodice led the way for women in medicine

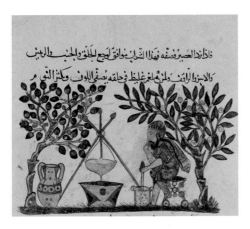

Cutting edge: it was through Córdoba that Arab medical knowledge flowed into Europe

Arabic. The chief physician was Jurjīs ibn Bukhtīshū, the first of six generations of doctor-translators.

At the beginning of the 9th century a rival to Jundi Shāhpūr, the House of Wisdom, was built in Baghad. In 830, a Nestorian from Jundi Shāhpūr, Hunayn ibn Ishāq, was put in charge of the House of Wisdom and translated many of Galen's works into Syriac and Arabic. Although the foundations of Arab medicine were laid on the Hellenic texts and the traditions of India and the Near East, Arab physicians and surgeons soon went far beyond these beginnings.

The first great medical school in Europe was founded under Muslim rule in Córdoba, so despite its geographic location it should properly be considered one of the fruits of Arab medicine.

It was through Córdoba that Arab (and therefore Greek) medical knowledge flowed into Europe. The first translations of the Arab and Greek texts into Latin, which made them available to the rest of Europe, took place here. And it was near Córdoba that Abulcasis (c.936–1013), one of the greatest surgeons of his (or any) age, lived and worked.

While Arab medicine flourished in Spain and the Middle East, the first European medical school was established at Salerno, Italy, in the 10th century. It was the outstanding medical institution of its time and it set the model for further Italian medical schools in Bologna and Padova and the great French medical schools in Montpellier and Paris. In 1221, the holy Roman emperor Frederick II decreed that only those publicly approved by the masters of Salerno could practise medicine.

As a result, scholars from all over Europe flocked to the medical school, including women (so there was no need for would-be Hagnodices to dress up). This was not unique: Muslim hospitals employed female physicians in the 12th century and female surgeons are shown in an illustrated copy of Şerafeddin Sabuncuoğlu's *Imperial Surgery* produced in the 15th century.

TOWARDS MODERN MEDICAL TRAINING

The medical schools brought a new type of medical professional to Europe. As we have seen (p.23), these institutions taught anatomy and they began to allow the dissection of human corpses. The model of the body finally shifted away from that taught by Hippocrates and Galen and came to resemble reality. Just as important, the model of medicine as a discipline changed, with the acceptance of past authority giving

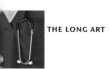

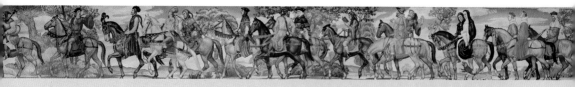

A 'DOCTOUR OF PHISIK'

The 'doctour of phisik' in Chaucer's *Canterbury Tales* was modelled on John of Gaddesden, an English doctor who studied at Montpellier, which took over from Salerno as the premier European medical school in the early 13th century.

With us ther was a doctour of phisik;
In al this world ne was ther noon hym lik,
To speke of phisik and surgerye,
For he was grounded in astronomye.
He kepte his pacient a ful greet deel
In houres by his magiyk natureel.
Wel koude he fortunen the ascendant
Of his ymages for his pacient.
He knew the cause of everich maladye

Chaucer's doctor, who accompanied pilgrims along the route to Canterbury, made a good living treating patients during the plague

Were it of hoot, or coold, or moyste, or drye,
And where they engendred, and of
what humour.
…
Wel knew he the olde Esculapius,
And Deyscorides, and eek Rufus,
Olde Ypocras, Haly, and Galyen,
Serapion, Razis, and Avycen,
Averrois, Damascien, and Constantyn,
Bernard, and Gatesden and Gilbertyn.

General Prologue to *The Canterbury Tales*, 411–34

way to exploration and discovery. This is the form in which medical schools have proliferated and flourished.

Exactly what doctors learn at medical school has, of course, changed over time. From learning the liberal arts, delivered in Latin, in the late Middle Ages, students have progressed to gaining a scientific grounding in biology, chemistry, genetics and pharmacology, as well as anatomy and medicine. The way in which medical practice was taught evolved only gradually, though, until the start of the 20th century. Then the Canadian Sir William Osler (1849–1919) almost single-handedly changed the system. Born in Bond Head (now Ontario), Osler

became one of the most important and influential doctors of modern times, laying the foundations of the present method of training doctors. Working as one of the first professors at Johns Hopkins University School of Medicine and then as Regius Professor of Medicine at Oxford, he placed great emphasis on trainee doctors looking at and speaking to patients. He insisted that students attend patients' bedsides early in their training and accompany senior doctors on their ward rounds. It was he, too, who instituted the medical residency – the period of time a graduate doctor spends in supervised practice. Osler died in 1919, during the Spanish flu pandemic.

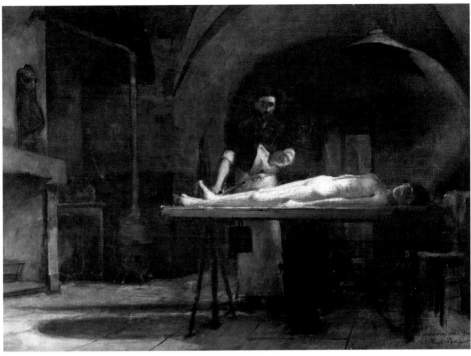

Dissection *by Paul Buffet: this 19th-century oil painting shows artists were as fascinated by the body as doctors*

VIOLENCE AGAINST VEGETABLES

In ancient India, Susruta trained his students for six years. During this time they had to practise eight surgical techniques: excision, incision, scraping, probing, scarification, puncturing, bloodletting and suturing. Surgical incisions were practised on vegetables such as gourds and cucumbers and on leather bags filled with mud of different densities. Students practised scraping using the hairy skin of animals and they punctured the veins of dead animals and lotus stalks. They probed rotten or moth-eaten wood or bamboo and tried scarification on wooden planks smeared with beeswax.

OUTSIDE THE MEDICAL SCHOOLS

While doctors enjoyed a university education, many other medical professionals – such as surgeons, nurses and midwives – did not learn from lectures and books. For much of history, professionals with practical skills learned on the job, apprenticed to someone already in practice. In 16th-century Europe, trainees such as the young Paracelsus had to demonstrate their skill in order to gain a licence to practise. And before Ambroise Paré became a surgeon he had to learn the trade of barber-surgeon from his father and uncle.

Training was not required by all cultures. The larger the role of magic, the more secretive, privileged and esoteric the initiation has tended to be. Sometimes,

OSLER'S PRANK – *PENIS CAPTIVUS*

Osler was a well-known prankster. One of his more successful pranks was the publication of a paper on the fictional condition *penis captivus*. Writing under the name Egerton Yorrick Davis, Osler published an article in *The Philadelphia Medical News* in 1884 which described a condition in which the muscles of the vagina could clamp so securely on to the penis during intercourse that it became impossible to withdraw the organ. The non-existent condition has entered urban legend, but there has only ever been one reported case, which was in 1947.

Sir William Osler was a medical all-rounder as well as a joker

medical responsibility was foisted on someone with no particular inclination to take it. In 1910, Walter McClintock reported on the method by which a Native American tribe chose a new medicine man. The elders of the tribe prowled around the encampment at night-time, with the ceremonial medicine pipe hidden under a cloak, while they looked for a likely candidate. The man they gave it to was obliged to become the medicine man, like it or not, because illness or death would surely follow if he refused. Being a medicine man was expensive and time-consuming, so some men would hide themselves on the night that the medicine pipe was to be bestowed. The new medicine man did not need to know much, because the medicine pipe held its own magic. Similarly, the Akikuyu tribe in East Africa traditionally believed that their medicine man was chosen by the gods. It was thought that the chosen man would have dreams that revealed his fate to him. If he did not tell others about them he would suffer as a consequence. He did not need training, because being a medicine man was a divine appointment.

Hospitals

Medical professionals do not always act alone: most are part of an extended medical community. Today, that community is vast – it encompasses a global network of hospitals, universities, research laboratories and private businesses. Over a period of more than 1,000 years, hospitals have become the main locus of medical care, especially for the more serious types of illness and injury.

TEMPLES OF HEALTH

When sick ancient Greeks went to the temple of Asclepius to sleep and hope for dreams, they were prepared first in the *kline* – a special sacred area, sometimes just an animal-skin mat. The *kline*, from which we derive the word clinic, is perhaps the first space devoted to something like hospital care. But this is small beer. The first dedicated hospitals were established in Sri Lanka in the 4th century BC by King

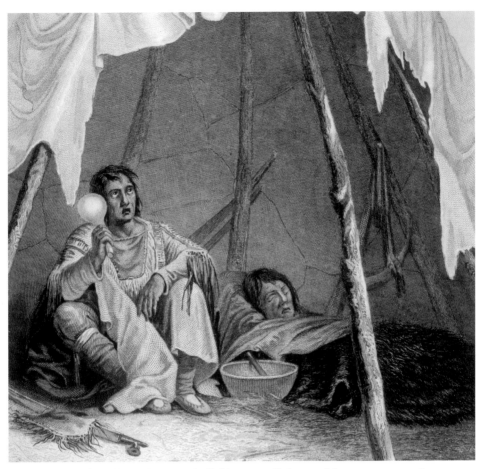

The healing arts of the Native Americans: inside his teepee, a Dakota medicine man treats a patient with medicine and magic

Pandukabhaya – they provided free care for the sick and lying-in homes for pregnant women. The ruins at Mihintale, Sri Lanka, are thought to be those of the oldest surviving hospital. They include a stone bath in which patients were immersed in medicinal oils. The great Indian king Asoka (or Ashoka) is said to have established a chain of 18 hospitals in Hindustan in around 230BC. There were even veterinary hospitals. A record from his reign reports:

Everywhere [Asoka] erected two kinds of hospitals, hospitals for people and hospitals for animals. Where there were no healing herbs for people and animals, he ordered that they be bought and planted.

The Romans built *valetudinaria* (military hospitals) from around 100BC in order to care for sick and injured soldiers, but did not provide general hospitals for the whole population.

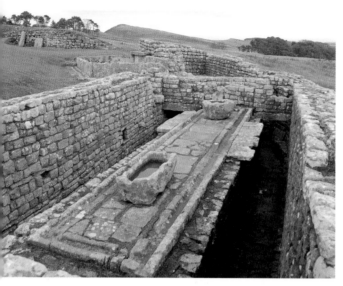

Housesteads Fort on Hadrian's Wall which boasted not only a valetudinarium *and barracks, but also a multi-seated latrine*

As Christianity spread through Europe, the requirement to act charitably led to the opening of places for tending the sick. These were not hospitals in the modern sense of the word but refuges, where monks and nuns provided food, shelter and medicinal herbs. They were often used for secluding the sick – that is, segregating them from society – but they were hardly centres of medical excellence and they were not involved in surgery, research or education.

THE GREAT MUSLIM HOSPITALS

The earliest hospitals that we would recognize as such were built throughout the Middle East, starting with Damascus in 707. These large public centres for healing the sick were called *bimaristans*. The sick were cared for by qualified staff, including specialists for different conditions. There

were wards for different conditions, too, so that those with contagious diseases could be separated.

Some *bimaristans* were very large: the 13th-century Qalawun hospital in Cairo had room for 8,000 patients. As well as physicians and surgeons there were nurses (some female), and pharmacists. These hospitals had their own dispensaries, teaching facilities and research areas. They were true teaching hospitals, with the training of new physicians as one of their main aims. There were not only hospitals for those suffering from physical ailments but also, for the first time, psychiatric hospitals, the first being in Cairo. The Arabs built hospitals in locations that were considered healthy, such as on hills (for fresh air) and beside rivers. When the *bimaristan* in Cairo was being planned, the site was chosen by depositing pieces of fresh meat around the city and then watching their rate of decay, in order to find the location with the freshest air.

Within a *bimaristan*, staff worked shifts so that there were people in attendance day and night. Once admitted, a patient could stay for as long as necessary – that is, until he or she recovered or died. Recovered patients were considered fit for discharge when they could eat a whole chicken. Patients were supplied with clean clothes and even pocket money on discharge so that they could convalesce before returning to work. If patients could not sleep, diversions

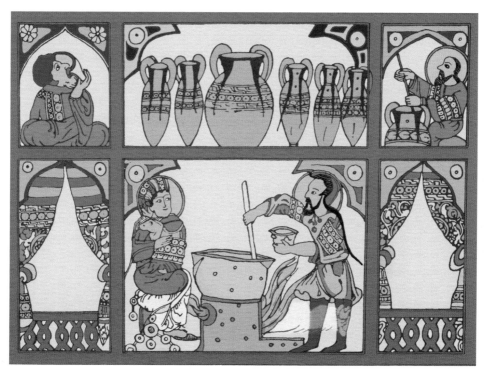

A Persian pharmacy of the 13th century: after the Islamic conquest, medicine continued to flourish in Persia with many advances being made

such as soft music, professional story-tellers and a library helped to amuse them. Healthcare was free for all. There was even a system of quality control to ensure that physicians acted in their patients' best interests. The contemporary writer Ibn Al-Ukhwah explained how it worked:

The physician asks the patient about the cause of his illness and the pain he feels. He prepares syrups and other drugs, then writes a copy of the prescription to the parents attending with the patient. The following day he re-examines the patient and looks at the drugs and asks him how he feels, and accordingly advises the patient. This procedure is repeated every day until the patient is either cured or dies. If the patient is cured, the physician is paid. If the patient dies, his parents go to the chief doctor and present the prescriptions written by the physician. If the chief doctor judges that the physician has performed his job without negligence, he tells the parents that death was natural; if he judges otherwise, he informs them to take the blood money of their relative from the physician as his death was the result of his bad performance and negligence. In this honourable way they were sure that medicine was practised by experienced, well trained personnel.

There were even *bimaristans* in prisons and mobile *bimaristans* that travelled to outlying areas in order to take healthcare to people who lived far from hospitals. The level of care provided in the medieval Islamic states was not matched in Europe until the 19th century.

EUROPEAN HOSPITALS

The returning Crusaders carried the concept of hospitals back to Europe. Les Quinze-Vingts, the first hospital in Paris, was founded by Louis IX between 1254 and 1260, after he had been on the Seventh Crusade in 1248. From the start, the hospital has specialized in diseased or injured eyes. In 1779 the hospital moved to its present site, and in 1780 the first guide dog for the blind was trained there.

European hospitals were often attached to monasteries and until the 16th century many of the staff were monks. In the early days, hospitals often had no permanent medical staff at all: monks ran the hospital, and doctors visited occasionally.

Religious ritual was observed and patients had to act morally. As soon as patients arrived at the hospital of St-Pol in

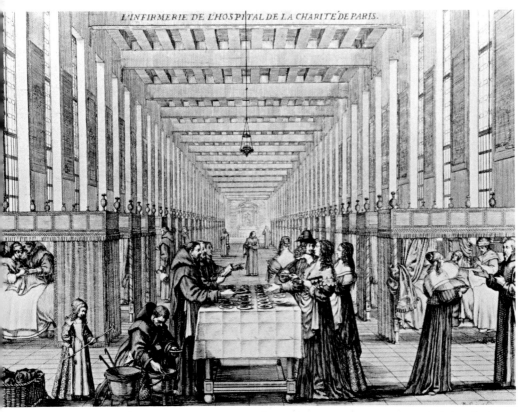

Monks and women attend the sick as meals are served at the Hôpital de Charité, Paris which dates back to the 17th century. The building was destroyed in 1935 to make way for the new Faculty of Medicine

France, they would have to take confession. Without it, they would not be admitted, just as a patient might be denied admittance to an American hospital today without proof of insurance. The medieval hospital did not want unconfessed sinners dying on its premises, thereby making the hospital liable for their eternal damnation. The sisters who tended the sick had to act morally, too. Anyone at the hospital of Vernon who was found guilty of sins of the flesh, for instance, had to lie on the floor of the entrance to the chapterhouse for 40 days so that others might 'step on her, like vileness and filth'. This did little to help the care of patients in the hospital, but a lot to underline its status as a religious establishment.

In Britain, the dissolution of the monasteries by Henry VIII between 1536 and 1541 led to the closure and asset-stripping of most of the hospitals. A few, including St Bartholomew's, Bethlem (Bedlam, see below) and St Thomas's (all in London) were re-established as secular institutions. But while the rest of Europe continued to build religious hospitals, there were very few hospitals in Britain.

By 1700, there were only two medical hospitals in London and none outside the capital. In mainland Europe, the hospitals were an uneasy alliance of largely secular physicians and mostly religious nurses and administrators.

In the 18th century, though, the spirit of the Enlightenment led to a spate of hospital endowment. Five new hospitals were built in London in the first half of the century and in 1729 a hospital was opened in Edinburgh, the first outside London. By the end of the century, all of

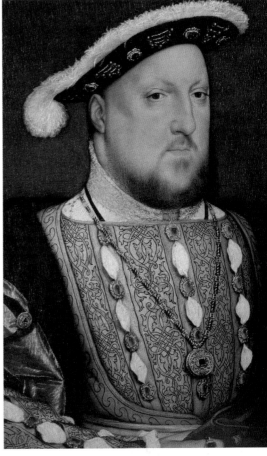

Henry went in for medical asset-stripping at the same time as he was dissolving the monasteries

the major English towns had a hospital. In Europe, Emperor Joseph II built exemplary hospitals all around the Hapsburg Empire, and Catherine the Great of Russia set up the immense Obukhov Hospital in the Ukraine. At the same time, hospitals began to open in North America. The first one was built in Philadelphia in 1751, and was followed by the New York Hospital 20 years later. Hospitals began to admit students, and

THE ALLGEMEINES KRANKENHAUS, VIENNA

The general hospital in Vienna, Austria, the Allgemeines Krankenhaus, was the leading European hospital in the 18th century. Begun in 1686, it was rebuilt by Emperor Joseph II in 1784, and followed the tradition of housing the poor as well as treating the sick. It had six medical, four surgical and four clinical sections, as well as staff training facilities, and it was designed to hold 1,600 patients. The hospital had the first dedicated building for housing the insane, the Narrenturm (fools' tower), which is a round building with individual cells, each with a slit window, a latticed door and rings for chaining up the inmates.

There are 28 cells on each of its six floors. The Narrenturm has one of the oldest lightning rods in the world. It was apparently installed because the electric current was considered good for the patients. The Allgemeines Krankenhaus was the scene of Semmelweis' work on puerperal (childbed) fever and Landsteiner's discovery of blood groups.

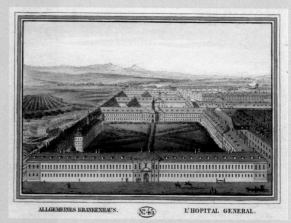

ALLGEMEINES KRANKENHAUS. № 42 L'HOPITAL GENERAL.

The original Allgemeines Krankenhaus which had its own currency for use by its early occupants

mainland Europe saw the beginnings of the familiar routine in which a professor makes the ward round accompanied by trainee doctors. The idea was soon copied in Britain and North America. Initially, patients with a fever were not admitted to hospitals, because the result might be an epidemic that could decimate the other patients. Later on, though, special fever hospitals were founded.

The 18th century also saw the opening of the first lying-in hospitals (maternity hospitals) where women could deliver their babies and take bed rest. In London, the lying-in hospitals were widely used by unmarried mothers who could deliver without question and then deposit the babies at the Foundling Hospital in Bloomsbury, where they would be educated and taught a trade. Unfortunately, the standards of cleanliness in the lying-in hospitals were abysmal and many women died of puerperal fever.

OUT OF SIGHT, OUT OF MIND

In Europe, many of the earliest 'hospitals' were little more than places for parking incurables and leaving the mortally ill to die. Pest-houses (for plague victims) and leper-houses could offer little in the way of palliative care, so they became a means of keeping the afflicted out of harm's way. They were dismal, hopeless places, where conditions were often appalling.

Another type of incurable frequently locked away was the insane person. Although the *bimaristans* had wards to care for the mentally ill, which were separated from the other areas by protective iron bars, Europe has had a poor record of treating mental illness. The famous hospital of Bethlem in London (known as Bedlam), became a hospital in 1330 and first admitted psychiatric patients in 1357. It was ruled by a keeper and the inmates (not called patients until 1700) were inhumanely treated. Often

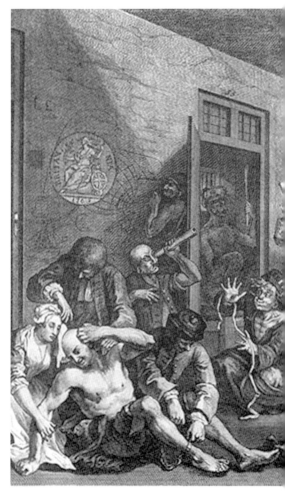

Patients were treated barbarically in early European mental hospitals – as shown by 18th-century English artist William Hogarth in 'The Rake's Progress'

IN THE LAZARETTO

The Italian diarist Rocco Benedetti described the old and new lazaretti in Venice during the plague of 1576:

But leaving the city and turning to the lazaretti, I say in truth that the Old Lazaretto resembles Hell, where from every side come stenches and intolerable stinks, the continual sounds of groaning and sighing. And at all hours clouds of smoke are seen spreading in the air, largely from the burning of bodies... On the other side, the New Lazaretto resembles Purgatory, where the unfortunate people in a sorry condition are suffering and bemoaning the deaths of their loved ones, their miserable state and the desolation of their houses.

kept manacled and living in filth, they were exhibited to paying visitors who were allowed to poke at them with long sticks to encourage their antics. Visits were free on the first Tuesday of each month, but cost one penny at other times. It was a popular diversion: in 1814, there were 96,000 visitors. Conditions improved in the 1860s, when the wards became clean and congenial and were decorated with flowers and bird cages. Though it has moved several times, Bethlem is still a psychiatric hospital. Even though the approach to psychiatric care improved in later years, brutal treatments such as lobotomy (removal of part of the brain) and treatment with electric shock were common in the first half of the 20th century.

The rise of nursing

While the *bimaristans* employed skilled nurses, elsewhere nursing was unregulated and often *ad hoc* until the middle of the 19th century. Before people became aware that cleanliness played a crucial role in the prevention of infection, nurses were doubtless a source of contamination. In Catholic countries, nursing remained in the hands of the religious orders, who at least had good intentions. Standards were uneven and generally lower in the Protestant countries. Nurses were often depicted as filthy, drunk and frequently cruel or corrupt.

The advent of modern nursing is usually associated with Florence Nightingale's work at the military hospital at Scutari during the Crimean War (1854–6). But nursing had begun to adopt a respectable face in Europe before Nightingale's revolution. In 1836, Theodore Fliedner revived the Lutheran deaconess movement, in which young women cared for the sick and the poor.

Prison reformer Elizabeth Fry set up a hospital in London based on the one at Kaiserswerth

He opened the first hospital at Kaiserswerth in Germany in the same year, where he instituted an advanced system of nursing training. The prison reformer Elizabeth Fry visited in 1840 and then set up a comparable institution in London; Florence Nightingale visited in 1850 and was similarly inspired.

When reports of the terrible conditions in the battle hospital at Scutari were published by *The Times*, it was Florence Nightingale who was sent to the Crimea to put things right. She took 38 nurses with her. On her arrival, she found that the injured soldiers were poorly cared for. They were living and dying in filthy conditions and were existing on a poor diet. Ten times as many died from disease and infection as died in battle. Cleaning out the sewage system and the hospital and ensuring a supply of good food and fresh air brought great improvements, even though germ theory was yet to be proven – Nightingale still followed the miasmatic model of disease. She transformed the hospital within a period of six months – in the face of considerable hostility – reducing the death rate amongst injured patients from 40 per cent to 2 per cent. The military discipline that Nightingale brought to nursing remained intact well into the second half of the 20th century.

FLORENCE NIGHTINGALE
(1820–1910)

Florence Nightingale was born into a wealthy upper-class family. In 1845 she outraged her parents by announcing her decision to dedicate herself to nursing. Refusing to marry, she became increasingly involved with Poor Law reform and humanitarian work. Then in 1853 she became superintendent of the Institute for the Care of Sick Gentlewomen in Upper Harley Street, London. It was from here that she went to the Crimea, at the request of her close friend the Secretary at War, Sidney Herbert. After contracting a fever in the Crimea she spent most of the rest of her life in her rooms in Piccadilly. During her remaining

The Lady with the Lamp: Nightingale devoted her life to nursing

50 years she was instrumental in restructuring health care for the armed forces throughout the British Empire. She also set up the first training school for nurses, the Nightingale Training School at St Thomas's Hospital in London, which opened in 1860.

In the 1870s, she mentored Linda Richards, famous as America's first trained nurse. When Richards returned to the United States she set up high-quality nursing schools on Nightingale's model. Although she was bedridden from 1896, Nightingale remained active in the service of nursing until her death at the age of 90.

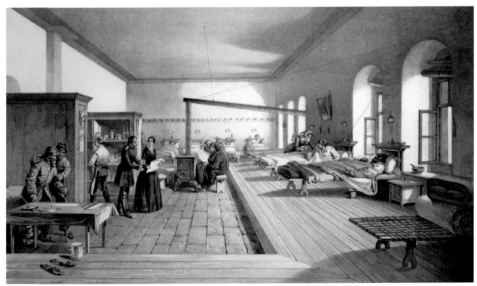

Florence Nightingale at the military hospital at Scutari: she went to the Crimea to improve care there

High-tech hospitals

Apart from surgical tools, medical technology is largely a product of the last two hundred years or so. The stethoscope and the clinical thermometer marked the start of the age of technology in medicine, but the advent of electricity brought the most rapid changes.

With electric light in the operating theatre and electrically powered machinery to deliver anaesthesia, surgery was revolutionized. Soon, machinery was

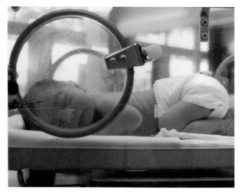

Protected environment: a premature baby in an incubator for the first few days of its life

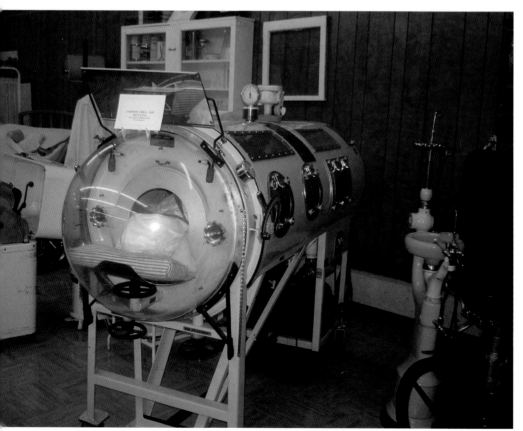

An iron lung: the patient may have had to lie in such a ventilating machine for many years, but it worked. There are still early iron lung patients surviving today

A CAT IN A BOX

Philip Drinker was investigating respiratory physiology when he discovered that he could accurately measure the amount of air a cat took into its lungs by putting it into a box and recording the changing pressure. Drinker also realized that he could reverse the process – he could change the amount of air in the cat's lungs by adjusting the pressure in the box. He gave the unfortunate cat enough curare (a nerve poison) to prevent it from breathing and then he managed to make it breathe artificially by changing the air pressure in the box. Next he built a large enough box to enclose a human patient. He tried it on an 8-year-old girl who had become unconscious after stopping breathing. She revived within minutes and asked for ice cream (which the cat had not done).

helping to keep patients alive. After the discovery of X-rays, it also helped doctors diagnose and treat a variety of ailments.

One important early innovation was the iron lung – a metal tube that works as a respirator. During the first half of the 20th century, polio was a common scourge of childhood. It left its victims paralysed and often incapable of breathing – many victims died. Then in 1928 Philip Drinker and Louis Agassiz Shaw of the Harvard School of Public Health provided a means of artificial respiration by developing the iron lung. Although it was initially intended for victims of coal gas poisoning, it became the standard respirator for polio victims.

Soon, hospitals throughout the developed world had entire wards dedicated to patients lying in iron lungs, some of whom faced 50 years or more of such incarceration. The iron lung continuously compresses and releases the chest by varying air pressure, like a bellows.

Modern hospitals rely on a huge variety of complex equipment. Machines now run intensive care units, replace or supplement the functionality of organs, image the inside of the body, assist in operations – the list goes on. The first instance of telesurgery – an operation carried out by a remote surgeon communicating with robotic tools using internet technology – took place in 2001. Surgeons in New York removed the gall bladder of a patient on an operating table in Strasbourg, France. With patient and surgeon being separated by a round distance of 14,000 kilometres (8,700 miles), there was a time lag of 200 milliseconds between the surgeon instructing an instrument and viewing the return video image that showed its execution.

Medical research

Many hospitals are now centres of medical research as well as teaching and treatment, but research has not always been so well organized. In the early days of medical research, some brave pioneers experimented on themselves while others experimented on hapless patients. The chequered past of medical research includes the heroic and dedicated individuals who often used their own bodies as guinea pigs and the unscrupulous experimenters who subjected others, often unwittingly or unwillingly, to new procedures and drugs. Slowly, more rigorous methods have emerged. Organized trials with control groups and monitored conditions have replaced earlier hit-or-miss testing procedures and medical ethics now protect patients. But the path has been rocky, and drug trials still go awry occasionally.

TRIALS AND TESTS

Long ago, the medicinal uses of plants and animals must have been discovered by accident or by trial and error. Potential cures would be tried out on brave or unwitting subjects. Some worked, some had no

Scottish physician James Lind conducted the first classic therapeutic trial in a bid to cure scurvy

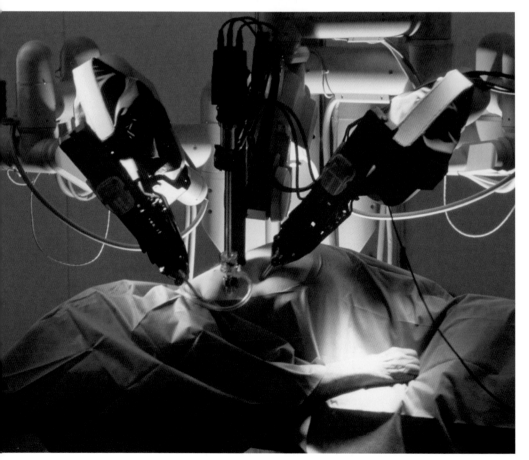

Invisible mending? The Da Vinci robotic system in use to perform laparoscopic ('keyhole') surgery

LIMEYS AND LEMONS

British sailors came to be known as 'limeys' on account of their consumption of citrus fruit. Limes contain much less vitamin C than lemons so they would actually have offered less protection against scurvy. But limes were cheaper because they were grown in the British West Indies, whereas lemons had to be bought from other countries.

nearly 50 years before the Royal Navy relieved the problem of scurvy by allocating a ration of lemon juice to all sailors. The actions of the Royal Society and Joseph Priestley had more influence on the decision than Lind's work.

THE SPARK OF GENIUS

Most early medical research was carried out by driven individuals, who often went to extraordinary lengths to test their hypotheses. Santorio Santorio's (1561–1636) investigation into the body's use of food involved weighing

effect and others must have made patients worse or even killed them. There was no way of predicting the outcome. The concept of any kind of comparative or controlled test did not emerge until the 16th century, when Paracelsus tried two supposed cures for syphilis before choosing mercury as the most successful. The first classic therapeutic trial dates from 1747 when the British naval physician James Lind was searching for a cure for scurvy. When he tried different treatments on each of six pairs of afflicted sailors, he discovered that those fed with two oranges and a lemon each day rapidly recovered. The remaining pairs were given cider, vinegar, sea water or sulphuric acid. Unsurprisingly, these 'remedies' were either useless or harmful. Although Lind published a paper that explained his findings it produced little impact: it was

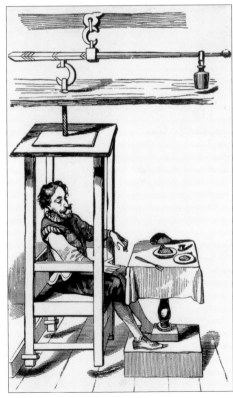

Santorio Santorio in the weighing chair he devised for tracking the workings of his own metabolism

197

himself and all his food, drink and waste products over a period of 30 years. Lazzaro Spallanzani (1729–99) swallowed packets of food in linen bags and then regurgitated them in order to study the process of digestion. Nutrition was an easy process to investigate through self-experimentation. The English physician William Stark (1741–70) lived (briefly) on a very restricted diet to see if it was possible: he died of scurvy after nine months, indicating that it wasn't. He worked out a series of 24 experiments to test his hypothesis that a 'pleasant and varied diet was as healthful as simpler strict diets'. He recorded the weight of everything he consumed and excreted, and kept a daily record of how he felt. After keeping to a diet of bread, water and sugar he felt ill after a month. He ate better until he recovered, then he resumed his experiment, adding one food at a time: olive oil, milk, roast goose, boiled beef, fat, figs and veal. After two months he showed signs of scurvy. He then tried living only on puddings, adding blackcurrants as his Boxing Day treat. Finally he restricted himself to Cheshire cheese, at which point he died. He was 29 years old. Unfortunately, testing fruit and vegetables featured later in his plans and he never got that far. More successful was Elsie Widdowson (1908–2000), the English

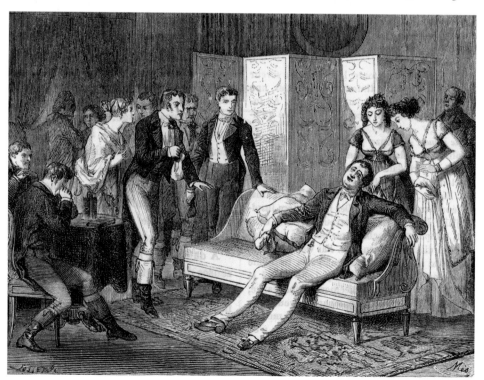

Self-experimentation: Humphry Davy became addicted to nitrous oxide (laughing gas) while working at the Pneumatic Institution, Clifton. He once inhaled 16 quarts in seven minutes

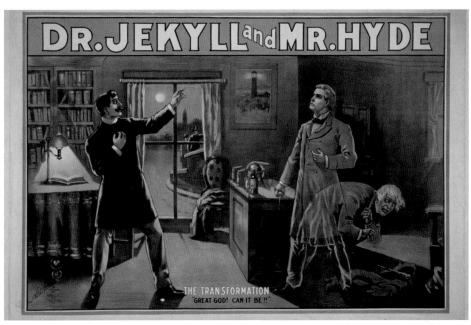

Dr Jekyll and Mr Hyde: *after injecting himself with fluid from the testicles of dogs and guinea pigs, Charles-Édouard Brown-Séquard became the inspiration for Stevenson's fiction about human duality*

scientist who developed the food rationing used in the Second World War by experimenting with her own diet.

Testing new treatments can be dangerous, especially when it includes contracting the disease to be treated. Compared with that, trying out anaesthetics sounds like harmless fun – the Scots obstetrician Sir James Young Simpson tested chloroform on himself and two assistants in 1847 and all three were found unconscious under a table. But it can all go wrong. Sir Humphry Davy became addicted to nitrous oxide (which he abused with his friends Samuel Taylor Coleridge and Robert Southey), American dentist Horace Wells (1815–48) was addicted to chloroform and American surgeon William Stewart Halsted (1852–1922) became

addicted to cocaine and then morphine as the result of his experiments.

Charles-Édouard Brown-Séquard only suffered disappointment when he injected himself with a fluid prepared from the testicles of guinea pigs and dogs in the vain hope that it would restore sexual potency. He was the inspiration for the fictional character of Dr Jekyll (and his alter ego Mr Hyde) and Serge Voronoff's monkey-gland treatment (see p.166). But how could the German doctor August Hildebrandt have been sure of the outcome when his colleague Augustus Bier injected cocaine into his spine in 1898? As it was the two doctors celebrated with wine and cigars when it worked.

Trying out some other medicines was dangerous and unpleasant. The 18th-century surgeon John Hunter reportedly took poisons in varying concentrations. Not only that, he possibly gave himself syphilis when he smeared pus from an infected patient on to his penis as part of a gonorrhoea experiment. No less brave was Gerhard Domagk (1895–1964), the German doctor who discovered sulpha drugs – he injected himself with an extract of cancer cells to see whether he would develop cancer. The German Werner Forssmann (1904–79) enlisted the help of a nurse to pass a catheter through a blood vessel in his arm and up to his heart. He then injected a photo-opaque substance and took X-ray photographs. Although his hospital banned his experiments on the grounds that such self-experimentation was unethical, he was awarded the Nobel Prize some years later. Another Nobel Prize winner was the Australian gastroenterologist Barry Marshall (b.1951), who drank a mixture containing the bacteria *Helicobacter pylori* in order to test his theory that it causes stomach ulcers.

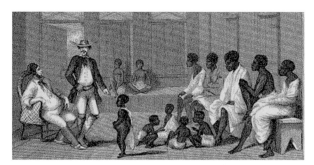

In the second half of the 18th century, the burden of supplying bodies fell on the less fortunate members of society, such as slaves

THE DARKER SIDE OF RESEARCH

Doctors are not generally encouraged to experiment on themselves, mainly for ethical reasons. But experimenting on others can be even more unethical. Following the explosive growth of teaching hospitals in Europe and North America in the second half of the 18th century, there was suddenly a need for more bodies – living and dead – to use in the training of doctors and the trialling of new treatments. The burden often fell on the less fortunate members of society. In North America, black slaves became the unwitting subjects of study in many cases – slave owners were offered the chance of sending their sick slaves to a hospital for a low fee. And poor people who could not afford treatment were offered free care in exchange for allowing trainees and researchers to practise on them. Some doctors specifically bought slaves in order to try out new treatments: a Dr T. Stillman of Charleston advertised for 50 sick slaves in 1838, clearly with experimentation in mind. In one documented instance, a doctor borrowed a slave called Fed to use in heat stroke experiments. On five or six occasions, over two weeks, Fed had to sit in a pit heated like an oven until he fainted. The doctor tried different medicines on him on each occasion. The experiment was reported by Fed after his later escape from slavery.

Not surprisingly, black Americans came to fear hospitals and doctors. Although the physicians generally aimed to heal their black patients, at least eventually, their treatment of them fell far short of the standards demanded by modern medical ethics. Black patients were particularly worried by the prospect of dissection after death – and with good reason. The shortage of bodies for dissection encouraged many medical institutions to dissect black patients, particularly slaves, without permission. They even paid for corpses that were taken from graves. Some black people prayed that they would die in summer, because dissections took place only in the cold winter months, when decomposition of the body was less rapid. It was not only black people who had cause to worry. William Beaumont's work on digestion was only achieved by forcing a poor French-Canadian trapper to become the subject of his experiment when the man had no other treatment options.

Secret tests on non-consenting subjects have long been carried out by military forces and governments around the world. Servicemen have been exposed to chemicals and radiation in attempts to discover their effects. At Porton Down in the UK, research into bioweapons included experiments on 20,000 human subjects, many of whom were not fully informed of what was happening to them. In the United States, the Public Health Service began an experiment in 1932 which, it claimed, would involve an experimental syphilis treatment. In fact, the subjects received no treatment at all. Instead, the research was designed to observe the process of their deterioration and death. Even after the discovery of penicillin, an effective treatment for syphilis, the men were offered no medication. The trial was halted in 1972 and President Clinton apologized for it in 1997.

> ### THE DISSECTING HALL
> *Yuh see dat house? Dat great*
> *brick house?*
> *Way yonder down de street?*
> *Dey used to take dead folks een dar*
> *Wrapped een a long white sheet.*
>
> *An' sometimes we'en a nigger'd stop,*
> *A-wondering who was dead,*
> *Dem stujent men would take a club*
> *An' bat 'im on de head.*
> *An' drag dat poor dead nigger chile*
> *Right een dat 'sectin hall*
> *To vestigate 'is liver – lights –*
> *His gizzard an' 'is gall.*
>
> *Tek off dat nigger's han's an' feet –*
> *His eyes, his head, an' all,*
> *An' w'en dem stujent finish*
> *Dey was nothin' left at all.*
>
> Anon

A TRAGIC TURNING POINT

The need for more rigorous drugs testing became crystal clear after the thalidomide disaster in the 1950s and 1960s. Prescribed as a sedative and an anti-nausea drug for pregnant women suffering morning sickness, thalidomide produced terrible deformities in the unborn child. Many of the affected babies were born with missing or stunted, flipper-like limbs. Between 10,000 and 20,000 babies in over 40 countries are thought to have been affected. However, only 17 babies were affected in the United States, because the FDA held up its approval of thalidomide for a year. The drug was only issued as an experimental treatment.

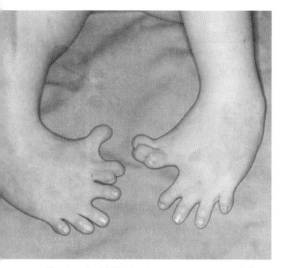

During the 1950s, inadequate tests were carried out on the drug thalidomide with tragic consequences for between 10,000 and 20,000 babies in 40 countries

There were suspicions that the large number of birth deformities might be linked to thalidomide, but doctors had not tracked down which patients had received the drug and then gone on to give birth to affected babies. It took some time to identify thalidomide as the root of the problem and withdraw it in 1961. Much of the detective work was done by two people – Karl Schulte-Hillen, a German lawyer whose wife and sister had both given birth to deformed children, and Widukind Lenz, a paediatric specialist in Hamburg. The pair drove around Germany showing people photos of thalidomide babies, asking them if they knew of any similar deformities. Thalidomide had been tested on rats but it had not produced the horrific side effects that were to appear in

STILL MAKING MISTAKES

While rigorous testing may avoid another thalidomide disaster, it occasionally brings disasters of its own. When eight men entered a hospital in London in 2006, in order to take part in the trial of a drug called TGN1412, six of them suffered serious illness. The other two were unaffected, because they had taken a placebo. All of them were healthy volunteers and they had been paid £2,000 each to take part in the trial. Within minutes of taking the first dose of the drug the six affected men fell ill. They developed pain, nausea and falling blood pressure. After being moved to an intensive care ward, they suffered a cytokine storm response to the monoclonal antibody, their bodies going into overdrive in

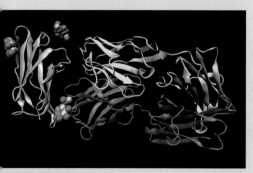

an attempt to combat the drug. One man spent 140 days in hospital, 14 of them in a coma. He developed gangrene, which turned his toes and fingers to stone and led to their amputation. The episode brought the ethics of testing drugs on healthy, paid volunteers into the headlines.

A computer model of a molecule of the drug TGN1412

humans. After the disaster, clinical trials became much more rigorous and in most countries drugs now have to be tested for effects on the unborn child.

After years in the wilderness, thalidomide is once again being explored as a possible therapy for a wide range of serious conditions including tuberculosis, rheumatoid arthritis, Crohn's disease, lupus, leprosy, macular degeneration, HIV and AIDS, as well as some cancers.

Medical ethics

The development of new treatments often runs into the thorny issue of medical ethics. It is not an entirely new concern. The first text on medical ethics was *Conduct of a Physician*, written by the Muslim doctor Ishaq bin Ali Rahawi in the 9th century. He described physicians as 'guardians of souls and bodies'. Gaining the patient's consent before undertaking an operation has long been seen as an ethical requirement. John Woodall, the 17th-century ship's surgeon, advised surgeons to obtain informed consent from the patient or the patient's representative before undertaking amputations, and in 1818 a Greek lithotomist using the traditional method

required signed consent from the parent of a young patient before operating.

In recent times the medical profession has had to tackle an ever-expanding range of ethical issues as medical technologies and possibilities have become more complex and advanced. Medical ethics is no longer confined to concerns about the proper treatment of individual patients. The whole of society is now involved in decisions about the type of research that should be followed or the medical procedures that should be undertaken. Religious or moral objections to particular areas of research are a high-profile example, but there are many others. We may ask ourselves whether it is acceptable for affluent individuals to harvest and store their child's cord blood (which they are unlikely ever to need) while public cord-blood banks are effectively overdrawn; whether organ donation should be opt-out rather than opt-in; and whether it is acceptable to help post-menopausal women have babies. Then again, how do we share out a limited budget for healthcare? There are endless questions revolving around our ever-improving abilities to deliver medical care.

Doctors are once again turning to philosophy, just as the classical Greek

---

MEDICAL ETHICS IN PRACTICE

Legend tells that Caliph Al-Mutawakkil offered the great 9th-century physician and translator Hunayn ibn Ishāq great riches to create a poison to use against an enemy. Hunayn refused and the caliph increased the price. Hunayn refused again and told the caliph that it would be a breach of professional ethics for him to inflict harm. Al-Mutawakkil imprisoned Hunayn and threatened to execute him for his defiance. Hunayn still refused to comply, whereupon Al-Mutawakkil released him from prison and rewarded him for his integrity.

medical thinkers did 2,500 years ago. Experts in ethics are being asked to give advice on which practices should or should not be allowed.

Writing tomorrow's history

The medical breakthroughs of the near future are taking place in the research laboratories of large hospitals, universities and pharmaceutical companies. They include greatly refined surgical techniques, stem cell therapy and drugs which target an illness or a lesion very precisely, with minimal effect on the rest of the body. Research into preventive medicine is directed towards discovering vaccinations against the remaining (and new) threats – HIV/AIDS, new forms of flu and some cancers – and ways of tackling the increasing diseases of a wealthy, sedentary population. We are still discovering things about the human body that amaze us. An experiment in Holland in 2009 investigated 'blind sight'. The subject was a man who had suffered a stroke which damaged the visual cortex in both hemispheres, making

DIAGNOSIS BY DOG

Not all new discoveries in diagnosis and treatment depend on high-tech equipment and drugs. Several research projects are investigating the use of dogs as a first line in diagnosis. The animals are able to detect the scent of some illnesses, even though no odour is obvious to humans. Dogs have demonstrated their ability to detect prostate and other cancers in some patients, for instance. There is considerable anecdotal evidence of dogs alerting patients to a part of the body that is found on investigation to be cancerous. So far, experience has shown that, if anything, dogs are generally too sensitive for the task. For instance, they can even identify which urine comes from which patient. They will need to be very carefully trained if they are to be used in the detection of a single disease.

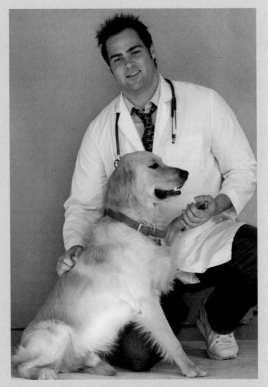

Healing hounds: in the future dogs could be trained to detect diseases in human beings

STEM CELLS GROW HOPE

Stem cells are cells which are at an early stage of development. As a result, they are able to grow into any type of cell. The most useful stem cells are thought to come from the embryo. However, the use of embryonic stem cells is very controversial, so ways of obtaining adult stem cells are being investigated. Because stem cells have the potential to grow into new tissue of any type, they offer the hope that the body might one day be able to repair itself. At the present time, the growth of new nervous tissue in spinal injury patients is being studied. It is hoped that paralysis due to nerve damage can be avoided or reversed. Stem cell therapy might also prove to be an effective way of treating Parkinson's disease, as well as some other degenerative brain conditions. Transfusions of cord blood are already being used to treat some blood disorders, cancers and diseases of the immune system. The first known successful cord-blood transplant took place in 1988: the patient was a 6-year-old boy with Fanconi anaemia.

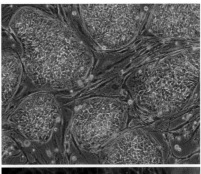

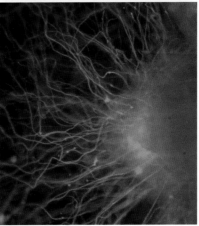

Our flexible friends? Human stem cells are capable of developing into many different types of tissue

him blind. His eyes were undamaged, however. In the experiment the man successfully negotiated a maze of objects unaided. Scientists suggested that signals from his eyes must have been transmitted to another part of his brain even though he could not consciously see anything. The body is still presenting us with mysteries.

Though humankind has taken huge strides in the last 150 years, the war with disease is far from over. New advances are quickly countered by rapidly evolving viruses and bacteria. Our crowded world presents an ideal environment for the rapid global spread of a new disease. The world's dependence on its growing army of medical professionals is increasing rather than decreasing. There is every chance that the story of medicine will remain a story without an end.

INDEX